LOVE
IS NOT
ENOUGH

A Mother's Memoir of Autism, Madness, and Hope

JENNY LEXHED

Translated from the Swedish by
Jennifer Hawkins

Arcade Publishing • New York

To my dear mother-in-law,
for all you have done for our son and our family.
There are no words to do you justice.

First English-language Edition

The author has changed some names for reasons of privacy.

Arcade Publishing books may be purchased in bulk at special discounts for sales promotion, corporate gifts, fund-raising, or educational purposes. Special editions can also be created to specifications. For details, contact the Special Sales Department, Arcade Publishing, 307 West 36th Street, 11th Floor, New York, NY 10018 or arcade@skyhorsepublishing.com.

Arcade Publishing® is a registered trademark of Skyhorse Publishing, Inc.®, a Delaware corporation.

Visit our website at www.arcadepub.com.
Visit the author's websites at www.jennylexhed.com and www.talarforum.com.

10 9 8 7 6 5 4 3 2 1

Library of Congress Cataloging-in-Publication Data

Lexhed, Jenny, 1967–
  [Det röcker inte med körlek. English]
  Love is not enough: a mother's memoir of autism, madness, and hope/Jenny Lexhed ; translated from the Swedish by Jennifer Hawkins.
     pages cm
  Translation of: Det röcker inte med körlek. Stockholm: Wahlström & Widstrand, [2008]
  ISBN 978-1-62872-429-5 (alk. paper)—ISBN 978-1-62872-471-4 (ebook) 1. Lexhed, Jenny, 1967– 2. Mothers of autistic children—Sweden—Biography. 3. Autistic children—Sweden—Biography. I. Title.
  RJ506.A9L49613 20115
  618.92'858820092—dc23
  [B]   2014035219

Cover design by Danielle Ceccolini
Cover photo: Thinkstock

Printed in the United States of America

CONTENTS

FOREWORD

All parents can empathize with anxiety over the risk of your child having a disorder. With being torn between wishing it were only your imagination and the persistent vague feeling in the pit of your stomach that won't be dispelled by reassurances. It may disappear for a while, but only to return when a new warning sign manifests itself.

In most cases, our fears are unfounded, but sometimes there is something that is not right. *Love Is Not Enough* is Jenny Lexhed's story of the creeping suspicion that their first child, Lucas, is not like other children. She describes the reluctant, difficult movement toward a painful insight. The book isn't only a story about the search for the correct diagnosis or the best treatment. It's about a parent's struggle to gain respect for her child from her community, despite all the diagnoses.

When I was at school to become a psychologist, knowledge in Sweden about autism was very limited, and the common hypothesis was that autism, in some vague manner, was caused by the parents' inability to embrace and bond with their child. When I read *Love Is Not Enough*, I think about all the suspicion these parents were subjected to. It's painful to imagine the burden of guilt that must have been placed on them, not to mention the feelings of powerlessness and vulnerability.

Theories about autism are being developed constantly, even though many questions are still unanswered. Some professionals still harbor preconceived notions, but many of us have developed a more nuanced view. We don't lay the blame on the parents anymore. Most of us have realized that the parents need support, even if support alone is not enough. In addition, many therapists have realized that the parents must be closely involved for the therapy to be effective.

It's hard not to be drawn into Jenny Lexhed's description of being lost in a forest of contradictory theories about autism and about the effectiveness of various treatment methods. For her, the never-ending hunt for knowledge led to a psychosis, which becomes understandable when you've followed her in her unrelenting efforts to comprehend, to put firm ground beneath her feet. Her weeks in the psychiatric ward are a nightmare in her account. Despite the fact that her depiction of her time there is free of anger and accusations—or maybe because of this—it becomes difficult to shy away from the huge shortcomings in psychiatry. The contrast between Jenny's ambition to put her son's needs before her own and the inability of psychiatry to listen to Jenny's own deep distress becomes heartrending.

Stories like this are critical for those of us who work in health care and education. They place the uniqueness of human existence at the forefront and increase our ability to empathize. That empathy is what gives us the power to develop treatments, support, and educational methods fitted to the needs of the individual patient and parent.

This is an important book, which can help other parents and families walking down similar paths. It will undoubtedly make it easier for them to find their way and help them feel a little less alone. And perhaps it will help them perceive the sunlight, even when things look very dark.

Per Naroskin,
psychologist and psychotherapist

PREFACE

TO THE ENGLISH-LANGUAGE EDITION

Love Is Not Enough is a bestseller in my home country, Sweden. It has been read by the mothers, fathers, relatives, and friends of people on the autism spectrum or with other disabilities, and by people going through a life crisis. But it has also been read by many others who simply treasure true-life stories.

I started writing because I wanted to put words to my feelings, to understand things better and make it possible to put hard times behind me. I took a writing class and received very positive feedback from my teachers, who encouraged me to publish my story. At first the thought frightened me, because I had really written from the heart and what I wrote is extremely frank and revealing. Would we want to share our life, our ups and downs with everyone else? Then I remembered that, when I first realized our son was different, it helped me a lot to meet other parents and hear about their experience. I figured sharing our story could possibly help others and maybe make their lives a little easier. So I decided to send the manuscript to several publishers, and three accepted it right away!

When the book was released, it received many positive reviews, and the media coverage was extensive. I was interviewed in newspapers and magazines, did radio interviews, and appeared on TV shows. From being reluctant to publish and share our story, I now had to face standing in the spotlight, which I wasn't used to and certainly hadn't desired. All of a sudden, I had to talk about having a son with autism and what it was like when I was committed to a hospital after suffering a psychotic breakdown caused by stress, exhaustion, and lack of sleep. This last part we had kept a secret, and only our close family knew. Writing the book, though, gave me the confidence I needed to stand up and acknowledge what had happened.

The fact that a few years had passed also made it easier. Our son was doing well, and I myself was leading a healthy life and working at our business. I wanted to show other people that it *is* possible to come back after going through tough times. The truth is, in the year 2001 I had an isolated psychosis due to a highly stressful life event in combination with a lack of sleep. Since then I have not had any relapses, and I'm not on any medication. I know, though, how important it is to lead a balanced life, and I always see to it that I get enough sleep (sure, sometimes it's less than it should be . . .), eat healthy, exercise, have time for myself and my friends, and most of all have time for my family. Having a loving family around me is a blessing.

After the book was published, I received many public speaking requests. I hadn't done a lot of public speaking before, and I wasn't thrilled about getting up on a stage and sharing our life. The first request came from the chief of staff at a mental ward. The hospital that had recently hired her was going through a transformation. Her background was in hospice care, and at her new job she was horrified by how they treated their patients. She wanted to incorporate the caring attitude that she was used to from hospice care. At the hospital, they had recently done a forced injection to a patient, and it had been an awful situation. She had read my book; she knew what I had gone through during the time I was committed and wanted me to come and share my story with the staff. I thought she was brave to change the way things worked on the ward, so even though I was scared to death, I accepted. If I could help the ward attendants, nurses, psychologists, and doctors to understand what a patient goes through and have them change their standard practice, then my fear of public speaking would be a small price to pay.

My lecture was for a small group of only fifteen people (which is much harder than talking to a hundred: a small group is more intimate, and you get much closer to your audience), but the lecture went well. The caregivers were somewhat hostile at first, because they thought I was just going to criticize their way of working, but they softened after hearing my story, and there was a great discussion afterwards.

That was my first public speaking engagement. From that day it rolled on, and over the years I have had more than a hundred engagements. I am of course far from perfect, but these days I have a lot more confidence when giving talks. One of my events was for an audience of nearly a thousand people and was broadcast on national television in Sweden. That was a challenge, and I prepared thoroughly for it in advance. I was, of course, very nervous. In situations like that, I calm myself by thinking of what I have that's best, and that is my family. Thinking of my kids gets me grounded and relaxed, because I know that even if I mess up and don't deliver a perfect speech, they don't care. They'll always love me, and that's what's important.

Besides having reached a broad audience, the book is also used in various educational programs and at universities, in courses like special education, psychology, psychiatry, and others. There are just so many things you can teach with facts, but reading about a real-life experience gives you insight that's priceless.

I receive many emails from readers and people who have heard me speak. Though I'd been hesitant at first to publish the book, I now know that I've touched many people out there, and I know our story has made a difference. One email I got was from a teenage girl. She had been committed to a psychiatric ward but was back home again. She had been depressed and wanted to end her life but now was feeling better and had read my book. She wrote that reading about my struggle gave her the strength she needed. She realized that she would overcome her own hardship and was inspired to fight on and keep on living. That email really warmed my heart. Another email I got was from the mother of a child with autism:

We fight, struggle, and argue for the sake of our kids. No one gives me the extra energy to make it through the day except, yes, my wonderful little daughter, whose laughter reaches way down into my soul. And my wonderful, proud son, who protects his sister at all times! And then there's your wonderful book. I bought it for all my relatives, and I'm giving it to anyone having a birthday. Through your words, they will better understand my life. Your story describes, purely and without varnish, what it's like to struggle for your child, to struggle until you go crazy, and then get up again and continue the struggle. Many thanks to you for taking the time and energy to bravely write *Love Is Not Enough*.

(signed) A Parent

I hope my book touches you as well.

Jenny Lexhed, 2014
www.jennylexhed.com
www.talarforum.com

LOVE
IS NOT
ENOUGH

HELP ME!

Can anyone help me? Get me out of here! I go to the light switch by the door again. I flick the ceiling light on and off, my only way to communicate with the outside world. I let it shine for three short seconds, then three long, three short: S-O-S.

When I've turned off the light, darkness sinks into my room on the seventh floor, my prison, Ward 22. I cross over to the window and look out into the dusky summer night on its way toward dawn. I peer out over parking lots, buildings, houses, and homes.

Is nobody there? Nobody listening, hearing, or seeing?

No one.

No one anywhere.

Just me.

Alone.

I rest my forehead against the cool windowpane, and tears run slowly down my cheeks.

HAPPINESS

Three years earlier, I'm sitting at my office desk, gazing over Johannes Park in Stockholm. It's early December, and the snowfall is light and flakey. It swirls slowly outside the window. A lone man passes by with his dog. A sudden pain inside my stomach, high up under my ribcage, is uncomfortable, and I move to change position. It's my first contraction, but I only realize that later on. I'm at the end of my first pregnancy. My baby is due in little more than a week, and I'm trying to finish some business and clean off my desk.

The office is lively. Telephones are ringing everywhere. People are answering them, chatting and laughing. There are ten of us working here now. The company is thriving, and we're being written up in the press. When we started out, it was just the two of us, my husband Carl and me. Talarforum is our company, our baby, in which we invest all our waking hours, from early mornings to late at night. In those early days, we worked out of a basement in Vasastan, a vibrant, fashionable neighborhood near the city center.

That was back when people still faxed each other, and the Internet hardly existed. We run a speakers' bureau and make our living on the spoken word. "Speech is golden" is our motto, in contrast to the adage, "Speech is silver, but silence is golden." We help businesses and organizations find the right speakers for conferences and courses. We seek out speakers who have a burning devotion

2

and desire to share their knowledge and experience, from politicians, CEOs, and experts to celebrities and performers.

I remember how Carl and I met just a couple of years ago: Moved in together, started a business together, got engaged, got married, bought a house, and now, soon we'll have a baby. It's all happened so fast, and it's been great. Sometimes I wonder what we did to deserve it all. Life can't get much better.

BIRTH

Lucas is born on a cold winter's day. It ends up being a long, drawn-out labor. The clinic believes that birthing should be natural, since there's less risk to the baby and mother. They believe it's safe to trust your body's own capacity to give birth. To ease the pain, they recommend warm baths, yoga, hypnosis, mental exercises, acupuncture, and TENS—transcutaneous electrical nerve stimulation—tiny electric shocks. In emergencies, they use laughing gas, nitrous oxide.

Early on in labor, the pain is manageable, but when it begins to feel too hard to handle on my own, I try TENS. It doesn't eliminate the pain, but at least I have something else to concentrate on—small, irritating electric shocks. After many long hours, the contractions ebb. The doctor doesn't want to wait, because my water broke the day before and the risk of infection is high. They give me something to bring on new contractions.

My labor pains accelerate again: strong, constant contractions, with no respite between them. It feels like my body is going to explode, and I fight the contractions instead of giving in and trying to relax. A succession of contractions wracks my body. The pain is intolerable, and I beg for laughing gas. I clutch the mask to my face, enter the clouds, and stay there. The gas makes me unaware of my surroundings but heightens the sense of pain, rather than dampening it. Finally, I can't stand it and ask for an epidural, but it's too late, the final-stage contractions have begun.

Forty-five minutes later (the worst forty-five minutes of my life), he is born. Lucas is blue on arrival. I barely get a chance to see him before they whisk him off, clean out his windpipe, and spray oxygen over his face. Soon, Lucas comes around, and I can hold his warm, soft little body on my stomach. He crawls up and finds my breast. A small miracle.

Is there anything softer than a newborn baby? New skin, soft and unblemished. I brush my lips over his velvety forehead and inhale his perfume. What if you could preserve that feeling in a little jar? A jar you could bring out and open from time to time, to remind you of life's wonders.

THE FIRST SIGNS

It's midday, just past twelve. People crowd the main entrance to the Åhléns City department store. Efficient businessmen and women enter the doors with decisive strides, running errands on their lunch breaks. There are people everywhere, but they flow smoothly and without bumping into each other, to the escalator that takes them up into the upper stories. Others stroll about idly, trying out perfume and looking at makeup in the cosmetics department here on the ground floor. Two teenage girls giggle with joy when a sales clerk helps one of them apply some eye shadow.

Lucas and I are waiting for an elevator. All the moms know that the best changing room in town is on the fourth floor of Åhléns. It is large and well organized, with couches to sit on and nurse your infant, several tables for diaper changes, toilets for moms and dads, a play area for siblings, and a microwave for heating baby food. It's on the same floor as the children's clothing department. When you've finished caring for your little ones and they're fed and satisfied, there's always time to look for some new garment they may need. The people at Åhléns know how to get parents to shop.

The elevators take a while. I see that both of them are on the top floor. Next to me is another mother. In her arms, she's holding a little boy with curly brown hair.

"*Hola, guapocito, mi cariño*," she addresses him in Spanish.

She kisses, cuddles, and teases him.

She tickles his ribs. He wriggles, trying to avoid it, nearly choking with laughter. Then he sees me. Maybe I'm staring, I don't know. My gaze meets his. He turns serious, his lips pucker, and I wonder if he's going to cry. But then he breaks into a giant smile. I smile back at him, and his brown eyes sparkle. He hands me his pacifier. It's blue and white, with a little brown bear printed on the middle.

"How nice," I say and hand it back to him.

It looks like he nods before quickly stuffing it back in his mouth. His eyes are still sparkling.

I turn to his mother and ask, "How old is he?"

"He'll be six months next week," she answers in broken Swedish and strokes his cheek.

"He's very sweet," I say, and she smiles.

I look at my own son. He has a tight grip on the edge of the carriage. He's just learned to sit up and still tumbles over easily. He seems entirely unaware of the little boy his own age right next to him. Lucas sits with his face turned away.

What is he watching? I follow his gaze. Maybe it's the small white table fan spinning on the counter over there, maybe something else. I don't know.

Ding!—my thoughts are interrupted. The elevator is here, and the doors open. People exit, and we enter. It's crowded. Two baby carriages, elderly ladies, young girls and men. A lady in a green coat stands close to Lucas. She smiles at him and tries to catch his attention, but he ignores her and looks in another direction. She seems disappointed. I watch the little Hispanic boy. He's smiling at anyone who looks at him, fully enjoying all the attention.

Faces don't seem to mean anything to Lucas. Strangers don't interest him at all. He's more fascinated with physical objects, like spinning fans or a fountain that sprays water, but also with shadows playing on the wall or bright lights. I think back to how, at his four-month checkup, I asked the doctor why Lucas didn't want to look at me or meet my gaze. She asked me to hold him close, turn him

7

toward me, and say something to him. He took a quick look and then turned away.

"There, you see?" she said. "He looks at you just fine!"

"But just quickly," I said.

"Don't worry. He's still little. He'll react more and more the older he gets."

She had no idea how wrong she was.

NEVER GOOD ENOUGH

It's nighttime. Lucas, who's one and a half, is asleep in his room, next to our bedroom. Carl and I are sleeping in our big double bed with Sara, our newborn baby. We bought the biggest bed we could find, so the kids would also fit in. It's more than six and a half feet wide and brimming with soft pillows and a couple of fluffy down comforters.

I wake up to Sara's small head searching and butting me. She's hungry. I give her a breast, and she settles down. We lie on our sides with our bodies close. I can feel the warmth of her. Her tiny body vibrates when she breathes. I caress her head. Her hair is so soft. She is four weeks old. I stretch for the alarm clock under the pillow and press the button that lights up the face. It's two thirty. I always sleep with a clock nearby. Lucas wakes up many times every night. It's important to get to him quickly so he can go back to sleep. If we wait too long, it can be impossible to comfort him. He can cry for hours, and nothing helps. I always want to know what time it is, so I know if there's any chance of getting him to go back to sleep. If it gets to be around five or five thirty, it's often better to let him get up. The clock also serves as my nightlight. If Sara can't find my breast, I can use the soft light to help her out.

Suddenly, I hear Lucas begin screaming in the room next door. I need to move fast. I nudge Carl, who's snoring beside us.

"Cut it out," he mutters in his sleep.

He's impossible to wake when he's in a deep sleep. Since Lucas was born, I always sleep with one ear open and wake up at the slightest sound. I give him a harder push.

"Lucas is awake. You need to go get him."

"You go, I'm asleep," he slurs.

"I can't. I'm nursing Sara. Get a move on before he gets hysterical."

Lucas's screams are louder and louder. Carl is completely out of it and doesn't seem to hear a thing.

"Come on," I say and pull the blanket off.

"What the f—?" he says, pissed off.

"You have to go get Lucas! He's screaming."

"Jeeesusss . . . Can't a man get any sleep? I've gotta work tomorrow."

He finally gets up, but Lucas is screaming to the high heavens.

"Try and give him some carrot juice," I say carefully. "It's on the table by his bed."

When I stopped nursing Lucas, we gave him formula. He refused to use a pacifier, so when he woke up at night, we gave him a bottle of formula to get him to go back to sleep. It turned into a vicious circle, since he woke up so often. Sometimes he would drink as much as four bottles a night. He had no limits and could drink until he vomited. When we weighed him at the children's health clinic, he'd gained almost nine pounds in four months and we stopped giving him formula. Instead, we changed to carrot juice, which he liked. He didn't drink as much, but it was enough to give his skin a yellowish glow. People would comment on what a healthy tan he had.

I'm in bed and can hear how Carl tries to comfort him. He walks around, carrying him, singing and shushing him, but Lucas won't calm down. On the contrary, he screams even louder.

Door hinges squeak, and I hear they're in the bathroom. Carl turns on the shower. The heavy jets echo against the slate tiles. I know he's steaming up the shower to make it resemble a steam bath. Then they'll stand in the dampness while the shower continues spraying water. The dimmed ceiling light shines on a pillar of fog in the dark room. Sometimes the moisture and heat have a calming effect on Lucas, but not this time. His cries ring in my ears. The two of them stand there for a long while, but the screaming doesn't stop. Then Carl wraps him in a towel, and they go out onto the balcony. The chilly September air surrounds them. Sometimes, the shock of the chill makes Lucas hesitate, quiet down, and forget what he was doing, but not now. The crying won't stop tonight. The full moon is high in the night sky and lights up the two on the balcony. I wonder what the neighbors are thinking.

In my mind, I blame Carl. Why didn't you get up when I told you to? Why did you wait so long? You know how he can get, how it just escalates.

After a while, they come in again. They go into Lucas's room. I hear Carl trying in vain to give him a bottle. I wonder, how can a child scream that long?

Suddenly, the bedroom door is thrown wide open and the light from the big Nacka communications tower shines straight into my eyes. Carl storms in with Lucas in his arms, their silhouettes are clearly defined against the blinking lights.

"I can't stand it anymore! It's impossible to calm him. Damn it!" he shouts and throws the bottle of carrot juice at the wall.

The juice splashes everywhere, on the wall, the bed, the nightstand. Sara wakes up and starts crying. She's already used to Lucas's cries but not to Carl's shouting.

"You're out of your mind!" I shout. "Why are you doing that? Now you woke up Sara too!"

"Here, take him."

He nearly throws Lucas down on the bed.

"You get him to calm down, then. You're his mother. You should be able to get him to stop."

Then he leaves, and I'm alone with two screaming children.

I pick up Lucas, who's crying so hard he's shaking. I put him on one side of me and hold him close. We stay that way for a long time. The kids scream, and I weep. Sara calms down after a while, and somewhere around early morning Lucas goes to sleep too. I lie awake for a while longer. I can hear the TV downstairs. Carl has fallen asleep, exhausted, on the couch.

We do everything possible and then some, but it's still not enough. It never seems to turn out right. It's undermining our parental self-confidence, and we feel powerless.

Carl's feeling of inadequacy, about not being able to reach Lucas, leads to frustration and is transformed into anger, which never leads anywhere. It just makes things worse. He often thinks I'm the one who's in the wrong, that I should do this or that instead, I should learn to understand Lucas so I can comfort him correctly. It's just that there's never a correct way to do it.

DIFFERENT

Lucas is small, only two years old, when I begin to fathom and admit to myself that he's different. It's difficult to say what it is that sets him apart from other children. Initially, it was mostly a feeling, an uneasy omen of the great grief that was to strike us. He is our first-born, and we had no experience of how a child develops and behaves in the different stages. Otherwise, we would probably have reacted sooner.

At the age of one, he could name some things and made an effort to say words when he wanted something, even if he sometimes used the same word when he meant different things, but now he seems to have lost what he once knew. He says almost nothing. It seems like he has regressed. If he wants something, he pulls me along and points to whatever it is. He points, but otherwise he uses no gestures to communicate what he wants to say. He neither shakes his head nor nods. He often gets frustrated and angry when I don't understand. He screams, kicks, and hits.

He often doesn't react to direct address and doesn't respond when we call his name. He can't do what we ask him, unless he can read the situation and understand what is expected of him. If I ask him to pick up a ball that's in front of his feet, he can give me the ball, but he can't go into another room and fetch a ball. We start to wonder if he might have a hearing problem. But does he? When I say, "Candy," he comes running immediately.

He has poor eye contact, except for a few occasions when he's highly motivated, like when he's playing chase. He can play that game endlessly. He's totally focused, and he screams with excitement when we chase him around the house. His eyes light up then, and his gaze is intense and follows our gazes.

Many other times, he is entirely closed in his own world and is hard to reach. He goes off and only wants to watch cartoons and animated movies. Pingu, a stop-motion clay animation series about a little penguin and his family, is a favorite that he watches repeatedly. Short, simple, and very clear little stories, with sound effects but no words. Lucas becomes engrossed with the animation and gets hysterical if we turn off the TV. He seldom sits still while watching TV but runs back and forth. He bounces and jumps with both feet, up and down. Sometimes he drives around in his red Bobby-Car, a small plastic car that he maneuvers expertly. He gets up speed and drives straight over the parquet floor in the living room, then makes a sharp turn, just in time to avoid the recliner in one corner, skids around, and drives back. He backs up and deftly handles his little car like no one else.

His motor development is very good. He began walking on his first birthday, and now, at the age of two, he has a good sense of balance. He climbs around and likes to balance along the back of the couch. However, he doesn't seek out physical contact in the same way other kids do. He doesn't like to hug and cuddle. If I'm sitting on the couch, he may climb up on my back, hug me from behind, and press his chin really hard against my head. If I'm standing somewhere, he may come over, take my hand, and press his chin into it, hard. He seldom sits still, and in his search for contact we become like two magnets that repel instead of attract each other, for his advances are hard and often hurt. Sometimes, when he's very tired, he can sit still for a while in my lap. These are short periods, all too seldom, but I take advantage of every chance I get to hold him.

He has a different movement pattern. He walks on his toes. He flaps his hands, holds up his fingers in the air, and looks at them.

He's fascinated by shadows and points of light. On a sunny day, he can stand for a long time staring at the white kitchen wall, following the shadows of the branches shaking in the wind outside the window.

Otherwise, he has difficulty concentrating. Like a butterfly, he flutters around. Stops somewhere for a short while, then flits off to the next spot.

He doesn't like to play with toys but is more interested in examining things. He loves to spin things. If he finds a toy car, he doesn't drive it over the floor, he spins the wheels around and around. Rings, coins—he loves to spin anything that's round. He can also begin to spin himself around. Any time, without apparent reason. When he does that, we try to stop him. Otherwise, he'll continue until he's completely dizzy and falls over.

He twines strings. We have wooden blinds in the kitchen and living room. He runs from one window to the next and twines the strings on the blinds until they're one big mess, almost impossible to untangle. In the evening, when it's bedtime, he lies and twists my hair into tiny knots that I'm forced to cut off. It's hard to get him to stop.

He also likes to arrange things in rows. His movies, wooden train cars—he makes a long row on the living room floor. And he likes to throw things. He likes to stand at the top of the stairs and drop things. Ball, toy, whatever, he watches it while it bounces down the stairs. Several times, he has tipped the TV from its table. He even throws things from the balcony down into the yard.

He loves water. He can stand for long periods on a stool at the kitchen sink and pour water back and forth between mugs and pots. With most activities, he tires quickly and runs away randomly, but it's different with water. We encourage his desire to experiment with food coloring, and he watches with excitement how the red drops dissolve in the water, or we may squeeze out detergent so he can stir it into a pile of suds that glitter in all the colors of the rainbow.

He could stay in the bathtub forever. He likes to fill it with bubble bath and blow at the bubbles until they fly up in the air.

He likes to pull out the plug and watch the water go around and around in a little whirlpool, until it finally runs out. When the last of the water goes down with a slurping noise, he covers his ears.

At the age of two, he's discovered the toilet and it interests him. He knows how to flush, and he likes to put things in it, and then flush. The flushing sound makes him cover his ears. I have to hide my earrings so they won't get flushed down. He often takes the roll of toilet paper, puts it on the floor, and pulls on one end to see it roll away.

He has never slept much. He stopped napping at midday early on, before he was two. He still wakes up screaming several times a night and has difficulty going back to sleep. He gets up at dawn, often around 4:30 a.m., and now the TV has become a lifesaver. A familiar movie will sometimes get him to calm down and even sit still on the sofa, while I lie and snooze next to him. I take the night watch since Carl has to work.

When we go to bed in the evening, we try to interest him in books, but he doesn't want to look at them and throws them aside. When we go to bed, I like to hold him, caress and hug him, but then he pushes me away. He wants to lie by himself, not next to me, close to my body. When we lie there quietly, trying to go to sleep, he sometimes laughs aloud for no apparent reason. He just bubbles with laughter, as if he's captivated by the sound of his own voice.

He's not interested in other children. If we're in the park, he doesn't notice them. Instead, he stands in the sandbox and splashes sand, or he throws stones in puddles, totally unaware of others around him. He can treat his little sister, Sara, like an object or a piece of furniture. If she's lying on the floor, he'll come over and sit on her. He often covers her with a blanket. If she's lying in his way, he'll pick her up, sometimes by the throat, move her out of the way, and drop her onto the floor.

He neither cries nor shows in any way that he has hurt himself when he falls. He doesn't come to us to seek out comfort or solace.

Increasingly, I understand that Lucas is not like other children. He has always been different, a little more difficult and more demanding than other kids, but now the differences are beginning to be so big that they're noticeable. Somewhere in the back of my mind, the word "autism" is spinning. I don't know anyone who is autistic and have no experience with autism, but I know that it's a communicative disorder. I get on the Internet and find the home page for the Autism Society, looking for information. I read there:

> People with autism have great difficulties processing and understanding information so that they can create wholeness and context in their experiences. They also lack the ability to understand and empathize with others' thoughts, feelings, and needs. The symptoms are usually divided into three main groups:
>
> 1. Serious impairment in the ability to create mutual contact
> 2. Serious impairment in the ability to communicate, and
> 3. Serious impairment of imagination, play, behaviors and interests.
>
> People with autism and autism spectrum disorders often have a different, extremely uneven intelligence profile and specific learning impairments. Studies indicate that one of the basic impairments, when it comes to learning, results in persons with autism and autism spectrum disorders not being able to empathize with others, not being able to imagine other people's thinking and feeling, in other words, that other people's behavior and actions are steered by inner mental processes.

A lot seems to fit Lucas, but Carl and I don't want to believe it's that serious, as terrible as autism. Of course, it is hard to establish contact with Lucas, but he doesn't have a "serious" limitation in mutual contact. He shows interest in us and likes us. He learns things; if you show him how to perform correctly, he quickly learns new things.

We speak with Lucas's grandmother, Gunilla, about our suspicions. She lives nearby, sees Lucas several times a week, and they are really close. She often babysits him and his little sister, Sara. She loves her grandchildren and is truly devoted to them. She immediately rejects our line of thinking. Lucas isn't autistic. He's so lively and happy. So full of life and joy. He loves to run around and be chased by us all. He does have a hard time speaking, but he isn't very old yet. The arrival of his little sister is a big change, and it's common that children regress a little, but they catch up again after a while. Gunilla has a lot of experience working with children, and we want so desperately to believe what she says. She suggests that we find a speech therapist if we're worried about his language development, and we agree to do that.

The Swedish health care system gives everyone who lives or works in Sweden access to heavily subsidized health care. The system is tax-funded. The care is of the highest standard, but sometimes the wait to see a certain specialist can be long.

In our case, the waiting period is very long, in some cases several years for each of the speech therapists we contact. In addition, it's mid-May, and many will soon go on vacation. At last, we find a therapist who has time for us in October. Maybe it's a good thing we have to wait. Lucas may mature and catch up. We're going to take the summer off to have time for each other.

The summer passes, and the fall arrives. Anxiety is a constant presence, pressing away.

Things are not getting better.

DISAPPEARANCES

I'm going out for the evening, and Carl is staying home. I've told the children I'm going out so they know. Before leaving, I make dinner for the kids and, when they've finished, I clear the table. The clock ticks on, and suddenly I'm in a hurry. I dress quickly, put on makeup, and then say goodbye. I hug Sara, who doesn't want to let go. She's one year old and clinging, but after a while she goes to her dad. When I look for Lucas to hug him before leaving, I can't find him. I call him, but he doesn't answer and I can't hear him either. I shout to Carl.

"Do you know where Lucas is?"

"Isn't he upstairs watching TV?"

"No, I was just up there."

I run around everywhere, searching for him, calling. Sometimes he goes down to the cellar to shine his flashlight. I check there, but he's nowhere to be found.

"Carl, I can't find him," I call.

"Where could he have gone? Out?"

It's a warm summer evening, and it's still light outside. We take Sara and go out to check in the garden. We check the playhouse, under the trampoline, and all around the yard. We have a small pool, but it has a thick pool cover that you can walk on, and it's impossible to fall underneath. To make sure, we remove the cover, and he hasn't fallen in.

Carl runs around the block and down to the park but can't find him there. We begin to get worried. Maybe he walked over to see Grandma, who lives close by? He's walked that road many times and could find his way there. We call and check, but she hasn't seen him. She goes out to look around her house.

Carl says he'll take the car and drive around to see if he can find him on the street. He goes out to the garage, and I hear him call:

"Jenny, I found him. He's sitting in your car."

Sara and I run to him. There's Lucas, sitting in his car seat in the back. He has opened the door, climbed in, and seated himself. He's sitting there in the dark, completely silent. He knew I was leaving. He either misunderstood and thought he was supposed to come along, or maybe he quite simply wanted to come along and went to the car on his own initiative.

In the summer, we visit my sister and her family at a country house they usually rent. It's a lakeside place near Strömma Canal, but the house is high up on a big hill.

My sister Charlotta and I are preparing lunch. Our mother is watching the kids out by the pool. I look out the window and can't see Lucas anywhere. He's not with his cousins in the pool. Lucas loves to swim and spends more time in the water than on land, but now I can't see him. I hope he's not on the bottom, I think, terrified.

"Mom, do you see Lucas out there?" I call through the window.

"No, I thought he was with you."

He wasn't with us. I run out fast and check the pool. No, he's not on the bottom. Could he have gone down to the shore by himself? I can feel my pulse quicken and fear taking hold of me.

"Mom, Charlotta! Lucas is gone! We have to look for him! I'll go down to the shore. Charlotta, can you check the woods? Mom, you stay at the pool."

I throw myself down the steep path, jumping over rocks and branches in my way. Close to falling, I regain my balance.

"Lucas, where are you?" I cry.

Good God, please let him not be lying in the water. Don't let him be drowned. It feels like my heart is going to explode. The path is endless, and I can't get down there fast enough. I start to get a glimpse of the water between the pines. I scan nervously, searching for a body in the water. I can't see very well—there are too many trees in the way. Panic grows, and in my mind, a film is playing in fast-forward. I see how I arrive down at the shore. I run along the water line and call his name desperately. I don't see him anywhere. Has he fallen under the pier? I throw myself into the water in shorts and a T-shirt and swim out. He's not there. It's deep out under the pier. There is a lot of traffic in Strömma Canal. The water is murky, and you can't see far. I dive down so that I can see the bottom. The deep, chilly water shocks me, but all I can see is sandy bottom. Where is he? Is he alive? I think all of this, and when I reach the shore, I hear Charlotta call:

"Jenny, we found him. He's up here."

I deflate. Thank God, he's alive. I return to the house. My legs are heavy. They feel like I just ran a marathon, and the path feels long, but my heart is light. When I arrive, Lucas is in the pool, swimming again. He's probably completely oblivious to the drama he has caused.

"Where did you find him?" I ask Charlotta.

"He was in Phillip's room. He'd crept into his bed. I ran to the woods and went over to the neighbors first, but couldn't find him. Then I began to look indoors instead. He was in bed, under the covers, nice and cozy, resting and enjoying himself.

We had been calling and calling, but Lucas doesn't usually answer when called, so why should he answer now?

SPEECH THERAPIST

The day arrives when Lucas and I are on our way to see the speech therapist. My mother-in-law is staying at home with Sara. It's a cold, sunny autumn day, with crisp, clear air. The trees are shifting in different shades of green, gold, red, and orange. Some have already shed their leaves.

We're silent in the car. Lucas doesn't usually say much, but I like to comment on what we see, tell him where we're headed and what we'll do. Sometimes we listen to music, but today we're just quiet. I've longed for this day to come but also feared the consequences it might bring. There's little traffic, and the trip to Stockholm South General Hospital goes fast, too fast. I want to remain in this moment, here and now. Pretend that we're just taking a drive, my son and me, without any particular destination. He is so sweet, sitting in his car seat in the front, turned toward me. He has short, blond hair that's a little unruly. He looks at me with his big blue eyes. His round face looks serious. Perhaps he can feel my mood? I take his chubby little hand in mine. He lets me hold it for a while, then he looks at me, smiles and says, "Mommy." I press his hand a little harder, and he pulls away.

We park in the garage beneath the hospital and walk in through the garage entrance. I show Lucas which elevator button to push, and he jabs it several times. In the elevator, he's excited and pushes all the buttons he sees. I just manage to prevent him from pressing the alarm button. We get out on the main floor and walk through the giant hall. There are many people in motion. White-frocked nurses walk around in their Birkenstocks, a young man walks on crutches, and a few elderly people sit in wheelchairs by the exit, waiting for the transportation service. A mother carries a crying infant in her arms. A stressed-out father pulls his five- or six-year-old girl by the arm and says she must hurry because they'll be late. I see a smiling man who holds a giant bouquet in his hand. He looks so happy. Maybe he has just become a father? Every time I step into a hospital, I'm struck by how much happiness and sorrow there is under one roof. I keep a hard grip on Lucas's hand. I watch him and feel a burning sensation behind my eyelids. Don't cry, I think, not now. We walk down endless corridors, take a new elevator, walk a little more and then we arrive. We take off our jackets and hang them in the closet. Lucas takes off his shoes and socks. He always does that when he takes off his jacket.

The speech therapist sees us right away. She's a young woman, about my age. She has long, straight blond hair that hangs down her shoulders, and she looks kind. She bends down, takes Lucas's hand, and says, "Hey, Lucas!"

He squirms loose and pushes his way past her into her little consulting room. She follows him with her gaze and smiles, greets me, tells us that her name is Helena and asks me to come in. We sit on chairs next to her desk. Lucas has already made himself at home and runs around like a whirlwind, picking up toys from the floor, throwing them, pulling out boxes and emptying them, pulling out books from the bookshelf. I try to calm him down and get him to sit in my lap, without success. He struggles, gets loose, and continues to explore the new room.

"That's okay," she says. "There's nothing fragile in here. We can talk a little while he's busy."

I try to relax, but I keep a constant watchful eye on Lucas to make sure he doesn't break anything or hurt himself. The speech therapist asks about Lucas, his birth, development, and family relationships.

She asks why we made this appointment. I tell her as well as I can. I brought his health records and she checks them. She asks about the BOEL test (a Swedish infant developmental test), if I remember it. I do.

Lucas was eight months old. He had recently had an ear infection but was well again. He sat in my lap, and the sullen nurse, sixty-something, was pulling out objects that he was supposed to grip. He took the objects and examined them but had difficulty giving them back again when she asked for them. Then she hid a little bell in her hand and rang it behind his ears. Lucas didn't turn around to find the sound, and she tried it again. He didn't turn around to find out what was making the noise that time either, though the nurse said she thought he moved his gaze with the sound and was satisfied with that.

Helena wonders if we redid the BOEL test, but we hadn't. She explains that the BOEL test was developed to discover at an early stage whether a child might have impaired hearing or other communication disorders. She sees in the medical records that he didn't babble at the age of six months, that he didn't understand words at the age of ten months, that he didn't speak eight to ten discernable words by the age of eighteen months or understand more, and that he couldn't point out the parts of the body either. In his records, it says that he's quiet and has his own made-up words. Lucas will soon be three years old.

"Can he make animal noises?" she asks me.

"No," I answer. "I don't think so."

"We can try later," she says. "Have you had a hearing test done?"

"Yes, at Rosenlunds Hospital, last spring. He has good hearing in his right ear, but for his left ear it's not certain, because it was hard to complete the test. I don't think his hearing is bad, though. He seems to hear well when he wants to."

She brings out a bag made of yellow printed cloth that reminds me a little of a gym bag. It has straps at the top that you can tighten. She tries to attract Lucas, but he's running around in the room, back and forth. I catch him, and we all sit on the floor. Lucas and I sit across from Helena.

"Look at this," she says and fishes up a small cow from the bag. "What is it?"

Lucas doesn't answer.

"He's not interested in animals," I say.

"What does a cow say?" she asks.

No answer. She picks up a car. Lucas takes it right away and begins spinning the wheels. "What's that?" she tries.

Silence. Lucas doesn't look at her, just spins the wheels fast. She takes the car from him, and he protests.

"Here. Take something else." She holds out the bag.

Lucas stuffs his hand into the bag and brings out a ball that he immediately throws across the room.

"A ball," he says.

"Ball," she says again, wanting him to repeat after her, but he doesn't.

"Take out something else."

Lucas retrieves a small scissors.

"Ma wha?" he asks and looks at me.

"Scissors," I say. Lucas doesn't repeat the word but continues to pick out things. After a while, he tires. Then she tries playing with him by putting different things on the floor: a truck, a cat, and a doll.

"Where's the cat?" she asks.

Lucas doesn't respond.

"Lucas, put the cat in the car," she says.

She continues with different requests, but Lucas does none of what she asks. Instead, he gets up, finds the ball, stands up, throws it at me, and says, "Owe!"

He throws it at me time after time.

"Hand," he says after a while, and he means that he wants to sit in my lap.

Lucas has developed his own language. When he uses one word it means one thing to him, but for us the same word means something else. It's as if language doesn't come naturally to him, and he tries to create his own structure and makes his own meanings for the words. Helena thinks we should book a new appointment for another visit. She has found it hard to make any kind of appraisal, since Lucas didn't actually participate.

We're back after a week. Once again, it's impossible to test his language proficiency. Lucas is restless, it's difficult for him to concentrate, and he shows no interest in her objects. The only thing he finds entertaining is throwing the objects onto the floor. Helena feels we should call it a day. I ask what she thinks of his delayed language development and wonder if she believes he might be autistic. She says she can't do an evaluation after so few meetings with Lucas but advises me to contact children's health services, which can arrange for an evaluation. She suggests the neuropsychiatric team at the Sachsska Children's Hospital. She also provides me with some informational material about children's speech and language development. Helena gives me a storybook and demonstrates how we can practice speech and language by reading stories. To facilitate language comprehension and expressive ability, she recommends that we use a lot of body language. She also says it would be a good idea to use signs as a support in communicating and shows me some different signs we could begin with, emphasizing the advantage in having as many people as possible in Lucas's circle use the signs with him. She advises me to read more about autism and gives me some tips on the literature.

Helena asks what our plans are for daycare. I reply that I want to be at home with the kids for a few years, that I'd hoped he would be able to go for a few hours each week to something called the church's Children's Hour, but that it hadn't worked out.

Many children in our neighborhood go to the local church's children's group—it's an opportunity for kids to play with each other and for their stay-at-home moms to take a breather. I had signed Lucas up because I thought it would be good for him to play a little with other children, so he'd get used to it before it was time to begin preschool. Besides, I felt it would be nice to have a few hours alone with our daughter, Sara. Lucas demands so much attention that she often winds up getting pushed aside a bit.

There was a waiting list for the Children's Hour, but I had succeeded in convincing them to let Lucas begin in the same group as Fia, a girl Lucas knew. Fia's mother, Camilla, and I had given birth at the same time, and we met quite a lot with the children. Since parents attended the school with their kids during the first week, Carl's mom, Gunilla, would take care of Sara while I went with Lucas. The children's group was held in an apartment complex. Two elderly ladies met us when we arrived. There was a huge room with a thick, red carpet in the middle. Along the walls there were lots of nice toys in different boxes and on shelves. In a smaller room next door, there was a low table with small chairs. The children usually sat and made things there, and that was also where they ate a fruit snack, explained one of the ladies. There were eight children, between two and five years of age. Several had gone there last semester, and only Lucas, Fia, and another girl were new.

First, we sat down on the carpet to have a gathering. All the kids sat down nicely, and the new girls sat in their mothers' laps. Lucas, however, didn't want to sit in my lap. He ran around and checked out all the toys. When I tried to catch him and get him to sit in the circle with the others, he screamed like a stuck pig. Finally, I got hold of him, and we sat down with the others. He continued to scream. I thought he might calm down after a while, but he didn't. He screamed and squirmed to get away. It was all very embarrassing, and I finally had to let him go. He went immediately into the other room, and I followed him there. We stayed in there while the others had the gathering and a sing-along. Then it was time for free playtime. All the kids began to play with each other. The new girls were a little shy at first, but after a while they approached the other kids. Lucas didn't care about any of them. He just walked around, picking up toys that he threw around. I tried to get him to concentrate and interest himself in some cars and a garage, but it was hopeless. I felt the searing looks from the ladies and the other mothers and was on the verge of tears. When it was finally time to go home, I was relieved.

We were about to leave, when one of the leaders took me aside. She said she didn't think Lucas was mature enough to begin yet. This activity only worked if the children could follow instructions. She pointed out that Lucas didn't seem to derive any benefit from the other children and he didn't even seem to know Fia, as I had said. I understood very well what she meant, but it still hurt to be told.

I tell the speech therapist that Lucas is on a waiting list for a Montessori preschool that his cousins attend. The children start there when they're three, and since Lucas's birthday is in December he has to wait until next fall, when he's three and a half. Helena thinks I should contact the municipal office and find out if there are preschools for children with special needs. I ask her to write an affidavit that Lucas is delayed in his speech development. I figure it can be a good thing to have when we do apply to a preschool.

Then we leave. I don't drive home, just around and around. I look at Lucas, seated beside me. He is completely calm, gazing out the window. I give him some pear juice, and he sucks on the straw. He is so sweet. He looks completely normal, like any other little boy. Could he really be autistic? Maybe he's only late in his speech development. Some kids speak really late. I've heard about that, and then, when they start speaking, they have complete language fluency. I want to believe that it could be true for Lucas, but somewhere I know it can't be the whole truth. It's hard to reach Lucas, to make contact with him. Sometimes it feels as if there's a thick glass wall between us, soundproof, as if he's living in a vacuum. We can't reach him in there, behind that thick plate of glass. Other times I imagine him being like mercury—like when you've broken a mercury thermometer and try to collect the quicksilver, and it just splits and glides away. That's exactly what it's like with Lucas. You can't get hold of him. He just glides away. Flows away. Disappears.

He gives me his empty juice carton. He's finished. Sometimes, he's almost like any other child and seems to understand and do the right things, but then other times he's so different.

I pick up the phone and call Carl.

"We're finished now."

"How'd it go? What did she say?" he asks.

"She couldn't say really. Lucas wasn't in the mood. He just threw things around. She thought we should do a neurological examination."

The words from my mouth sound hard, terrible and completely awful. "Then let's do it," says Carl. "We can't wait any longer."

"I think he's autistic," I say.

"You don't know that. He doesn't have to be."

"She said I should read up on autism. She said we should find out if there are special preschools in our town," I say, and I feel I can't produce any more words. My voice just stops.

I can't talk more now, and I hang up. Tears are running down my face. Carl calls back, but I can't answer. Tears are blinding me, and I can't see the road. Where are we? Where are we headed? I don't know. We've just been driving around and around. I cry all the way home. Sometimes I cast a sidelong glance at Lucas. He doesn't seem to notice that I'm sad, and I hope he doesn't understand. I don't want him to know I'm crying because of him, because he isn't like all the other kids. I love him anyway, as he is. Nothing in the world can change that.

NO TIME TO LOSE

Now we're beginning to feel there's no time to lose.

We're in a hurry to move on, to get advice, so we can understand what we need to do to help Lucas. I call the neuropsychiatric team at Sachsska Children's Hospital to find out if we can get him examined. I explain the situation: we've been waiting for a long time for Lucas to speak, and we've seen a speech therapist; she believes we should get a thorough examination and evaluation as soon as possible, since Lucas is very late in speaking and in his social development. I say that we'd like to get started with the process before Christmas, since we're planning on enrolling Lucas in a preschool next fall. We had planned for him to start in a regular preschool but are not sure if it would work out. Lucas may need another kind of childcare, more adapted to his needs.

I hear the nurse almost laughing at me.

"An evaluation before Christmas? It's already October. Sorry, there's a two-year waiting list to have those evaluations done. First off, we need a referral from your pediatrician before we can put him on our waiting list. Start by visiting your children's clinic."

A two-year waiting list? I can't believe my ears. What happened to the Swedish health care guarantee? Aren't you supposed to see a doctor within ninety days from the date you seek help? This is a little boy who needs help—and he has to wait for two years! I can feel panic rising. We can't wait two years. Lucas will be five by then. What if he has some kind of disease? Something genetic, that demands medical treatment? . . . I've heard of terrible diseases where children are born seemingly healthy, then just regress and sometimes die if they don't get help in time. What if he has something like that? Maybe he has cancer. Maybe he has a brain tumor that's keeping him from developing the way he should. He needs help now, not in two years.

"Is there any other hospital we can turn to?" I ask, upset.

She answers that there aren't many hospitals that do this type of evaluation, and she thinks that the waiting periods are just as long for them, but she gives me the names of some. I call around, but it's the same everywhere. Waiting lists. One nurse mentions that you can do a private evaluation. She has heard that Tore Duvner, a specialist in child psychiatry, now has a private clinic and does these kinds of tests. I wonder if she knows how I can reach him, and she replies that she thinks he lives and works in Nacka, which is close to Stockholm.

I call Carl and tell him what I've found out. He is just as upset as I am.

"That's outrageous! Small children waiting for so long to get a diagnosis. No way. I think we should have a private examination. No matter what it costs. We can get a loan if we have to. We can't wait for two years. That's intolerable. Are we supposed to just wait around and watch how Lucas is not developing, not knowing how to help him?" he says.

I succeed in reaching Tore Duvner, the doctor mentioned by the nurse I spoke with. As she said, he does these sorts of evaluations and has a three-month waiting list. He tells me that the evaluation consists of conversations with him, where he meets Lucas and us and, after that, they also do extensive psychological testing, including an analysis of Lucas's speech and language development. The tests themselves are not performed by Dr. Duvner but by psychologists and speech therapists he collaborates with. Somehow, I convince him that we need to start sooner than the three months. He makes the arrangements so we can start the various tests simultaneously and speed up the evaluation process. In one month, we can begin the testing, and the whole evaluation will be finished within three months.

For more than six months, we've been worried about Lucas. We've been waiting and hoping for some change—for a miracle. Now we've accepted that there really is a problem, we weren't just imagining things, and Lucas really is late in his development. The speech therapist confirmed our worst suspicions and fears. Lucas is late enough that we must have a neurological examination done. Maybe he has brain damage or a neurological disease or something else horrendous. I'm heartbroken. We ought to be able to do something while we wait for the tests. One month is a long time to wait when we've already waited so long.

I call the children's autism center. All the qualified people are gathered there: psychologists, speech therapists, and special education consultants. They plan training programs for autistic children. I ask if we can get help, but they say a child needs to be diagnosed before they can see him. Once we have a diagnosis, we can apply for their services, but they have also a waiting list, of course. One year is the current wait time. Children could grow up before they got any help at all, if they have to wait in all these lines!

However, they do tell me about a lekotek—a "play library"— and datatek—a "computer library"—that we can apply to if we have a referral from a speech therapist. I contact the lekotek and the computer resource center, and they also have long waiting lists, but I say we're flexible and can come at any time if they have a cancellation. I call them every morning and ask about cancellations, and within the space of a couple of weeks we have an appointment.

The lekotek is a resource center and lending library for special needs children. Families with "differently abled" preschool children can go there for help. We get an appointment, and a woman on staff does a learning ability assessment of Lucas, then advises me how we can stimulate his development through play with different learning tools and adapted toys that we can borrow and take home. There are simple games and small cars and airplanes that shoot away when you press a button. We borrow a sturdy tricycle, so Lucas can learn to ride it.

Lucas and I also visit the datatek, where he can try out different computer games. The datatek is designed for children and adults with special needs. Lucas likes it when things happen on the screen. He quickly learns to use the different buttons and then the mouse. The instructor explains how Lucas can develop motor and sensory ability, imagination, language, and concepts by playing the various games, and we borrow a couple to take home.

There is much more that must be planned and done. Lucas is to begin preschool in the fall. We have been promised a spot at the school his cousins attend, but the staff is unaware of Lucas's problems. Well, they know at least that he's a little late in his speech development, but no more than that. Maybe now they won't accept him, like the church preschool. Maybe he won't fit into their group and activities. Will he need to go to a special needs school? It all feels very strange. I call around and chart out what kinds of facilities there are for children with late language development.

I call the city, but they have little to offer. There is a daycare center where they place all the handicapped kids. Kids with autism, ADHD, Down's syndrome, cerebral palsy, and kids with various developmental disorders all attend. I figure it can't be a good idea to put all the kids who have problems in the same place. It must be incredibly difficult to achieve a quality activity that suits everybody, when the children have such different needs. Besides, I don't see Lucas as being handicapped, only developmentally delayed. Yet there is no special school for language development.

I call the speech therapist, Helena, and ask if she knows of any speech and language daycares. She knows of a few in the Stockholm area.

None of them is nearby. Yes, there's one, but when I call them and ask, there is a several-year-long waiting list. The closest, the Lidingö Home, is on the island of Lidingö, and it can take an hour to drive there in traffic. Then there's something called Hällsbo School, in Sigtuna, which is north of Stockholm. We can't send Lucas that far.

I call the Lidingö Home to ask about their activities. The Red Cross runs it. They have twelve children, all with serious language disorders. There could possibly be a spot open in the fall. We can come for a visit, and they want to meet Lucas to see if he fits in. The woman I speak with emphasizes the fact that they only accept children with language disorders. They don't take kids with autism spectrum disorders. I'm immediately worried that Lucas won't fit in, but I sign us up and we make an appointment to visit the preschool. If we're interested in the school, they'll meet with Lucas and do a developmental assessment.

Amid all this, there's everyday life. It's getting dark out now, and the days are shorter. Lucas will be three in early December. Relatives ask us what he wants for his birthday.

"I don't' know," I answer.

What do you give a child who isn't interested in toys, who thinks the ribbons on the packages are more fun than the contents? Lucas's grandmother showers him with toys that never get used. Lucas's room looks like a toy shop. Everything is neatly stowed in rows on the shelves or lying unused in boxes. Someday, I hope they'll be useful and that he'll want to play like other children.

December comes swiftly. Suddenly it's December 13, St. Lucia Day, almost a holiday in Sweden, with processions of white-clad girls and boys, wearing crowns of candles and singing in almost every school, daycare, and preschool. We are celebrating at home. There is a group of us stay-at-home moms, and we take turns hosting each other. I have bought soft red Santa Claus outfits for the kids. Lucas is extremely sensitive about the clothes he wants to wear. It's dark outside, and I've lit a fire in the fireplace. It spreads a warm glow in the living room. In the light of the outdoor lantern, I see snow-flakes slowly sifting down between the neighboring houses. In the background, I hear Christmas music. The moms chatter, and the kids are playing. Sometimes there's a controversy about toys, but nothing's impossible to resolve. All the kids play together and are having fun. All except Lucas.

I look upstairs and find him there. He's sitting alone, watching an animated movie. He has taken off the red suit and is sitting naked on the blue-and-white-striped sofa. I take out some other comfortable clothes I know he approves of, but he refuses to get dressed. I try to lure him downstairs, but he won't go. After a while, I give up and go downstairs to the others. I want to be able to enjoy Sara, who has fun playing with the others. Sara is sixteen months old now, and it's her first real Lucia, the first one she's old enough to experience. Last year, she was only a few months old and was mostly asleep.

She's so cute, running around like a little Santa's helper. A spirited, open little girl, who loves to be with the bigger kids. She is Lucas's opposite. How can siblings be so different?

The speech therapist advised me to read up about autism, so in the evening, when the children are asleep, I go up to the attic. We have an office in the attic, since Carl often works from home at night. I sit in front of the computer, search the Internet, and read everything I can find about language disorders and autism. The Internet is an endless source of information, and I want to read it all. There are no limits. One page leads to another. I sit reading for hours. I'm increasingly convinced that Lucas is autistic.

I mention my suspicions to Carl, but he won't really listen. He doesn't want to jump to hasty conclusions and prefers to wait and hear what the examinations reveal. As I read the specialist literature and become truly informed on the subject, though, I begin to be more certain that Lucas has autism—an incurable, life-long handicap.

I read everything I can get hold of. About what autism is and why it occurs. I want to know what autistic kids are like, how they live, the prospects for them when they're older and grown up. What kinds of treatments are there and methods of instruction? I read and read, and seek more and more information, tears streaming down my cheeks.

The tears never stop. So many dismal pictures are being painted. I read parents' tales describing everyday life with their autistic kids, about all the hopelessness when help is nowhere to be found, about kids who never learn to speak, who suffer from self-abusive behavior and whom no one has the energy to take care of, and finally, who often end up in institutions.

I read several horrible stories about how these children, who cannot communicate, suffer abuse in these institutions. In a British newspaper, I read an article about a single mom who couldn't take it anymore and committed suicide, taking her son's life too, by jumping off a cliff.

I read about Freja, a woman in her forties, who has been called Sweden's most dangerous woman. When she was little, she refused to speak, didn't want to play with other children, didn't like changes, and could, quite suddenly and unexpectedly, break things. She was taken from her parents, locked up, punished, and when nothing else helped, was given antipsychotic drugs. She was so badly treated she became aggressive to her caretakers. Not until she was an adult did a doctor realize she was autistic. After that, she received help, but her life was mostly destroyed already.

Until the late 1980s, it was believed that the term "autism" described emotional disorders in children that were caused by callous, frigid mothers. Psychodynamic therapies were developed to "cure" autism. Bruno Bettelheim was an advocate of this, and his theory was that the parents—consciously or unconsciously—harbored a death wish regarding their child, and the most important thing to do was to separate children from their parents. Today, autism is seen as a neurological disorder, but I read that there are still some child psychotherapists who believe the parents are guilty of a relationship disorder and are responsible for their child's handicap.

I picture worst-case scenarios. I imagine how Lucas won't fit in anywhere; in the end he'll be locked up in an institution where he's misunderstood and maybe even abused. That must not happen. Lucas needs help, but how could we risk leaving him with anyone? What do those people know about the latest research findings? What if they're stuck in the old ways of thinking? We have to do something. We don't have a choice. We need to make sure that our son has a good life, and we're going to succeed, no matter how dark things look now.

Slowly but surely, sorrow knocks on the door. We don't want to open it, and try to keep the door shut. We make an effort to live as normal a life as possible, at the same time as we're beginning to understand that our secure little world is falling apart. Maybe it never existed. Maybe it was just an illusion. Maybe we've only been living in a make-believe world, thinking it was fine. We wanted two children close in age so they could grow up, play together, and have fun with each other. Will they ever feel the joy of that?

What will become of Lucas? Will his speech ever develop? Will he be able to communicate with others? Share experiences and thoughts? Will he have any friends, or will he always be alone? Will he fall in love and feel the joy of being close to another person? Will he be able to have a family? Or will it be like this for the rest of his life? What happens after we die? Who will take care of Lucas? No one cares about him and loves him the way we do. My thoughts are spinning.

Sometimes during the day, I can't hold it back and my sorrow wants to take over. Like a hurricane, it blows the door wide open and the blackest sorrow completely
    rushes in
    washes over me
    drenches me.
Then I take the kids, put them in the car, and drive. I drive out to the deserted streets in the quiet, green parts of Stockholm. Sara falls asleep in the front seat. Lucas sits in back and looks out the window. We go slowly. I can't drive fast while my tears are pouring out. I cry until I'm shaking. I just want to shout. I turn up the volume on the radio, and the music drowns my sobbing, while Lucas sits in the back seat, apparently unaffected, staring out the window.

PLAN OF ACTION

Everything I read mentions how important early intervention is. The younger the child, the better the chances that therapies will be successful and lead to the possibility of a normal life.

I search desperately for treatments that might help Lucas. There is a wide variety of therapies: swimming with dolphins, diets, medicines, music therapy, audio exercises, tactile stimulation, behavioral therapy, and special teaching methods to communicate through the use of images. Some of them sound like pure charlatanism, and that's most often true with those therapies that claim to *cure* autism.

We know it will take time to get Lucas into the autism center where he can get help and we can begin to develop a strategy. We may have to wait as long as a year. Just like all other parents, we want to create the best conditions for our child so he can live as normal and rich a life as possible. Lucas just needs more help than other kids. We want to give him the possibility of a life without limitations. We want to give Lucas everything that Sara gets. We can't wait a whole year to get help, if waiting will decrease his quality of life and limit his development. We have to do something *now!*

I order more material and read everything, plowing through research papers night after night. Carl still can't really accept all this, but I cannot wait for him to understand. I take in the facts, assess, and slowly begin to build an idea of which strategies I believe in.

I talk with Carl, plead, and try to convey all the information I've absorbed. He has wanted to keep his sorrow at a distance. Slowly, slowly, a little at a time, it sinks in. His repressed emotions well up, then the sobs come, and we cry together.

I fashion a plan of action, establishing goals and the means to achieve them:

GOALS
Get Lucas to
communicate with gestures, signs, images, and speech
be able to sit and do exercises for a while, like doing puzzles, drawings, working with Play-Doh
be able to follow instructions
get dressed by himself
set and clear the dinner table
be able to play with toys
be happy and feel loved

MEANS
introduce pictures together with amplified body language
work with video to learn new things
work with computers
do exercises aimed at learning about colors and shapes
do things that Lucas likes to do: swimming, playing tag, and wrestling
be together with other children in groups
let Lucas, together with Sara, be the focal point

Carl is the CEO of our company and is gone every day until late in the evening. I'm at home with our two children. Sara is one and a half, and Lucas is three. There is a lot that needs to be done besides Lucas's training, like the laundry, cleaning, changing diapers, cooking, and making sure Sara has her midday nap. My mother-in-law, Gunilla, is there at my side. She doesn't share my view that Lucas could be autistic, but she realizes that he needs to practice in order to make headway with communication skills.

We need to help our child now. There's no time for tears. Lucas is the one who needs to be the center of attention, not us and our sorrow. I bring out materials and begin developing a method. Lucas has a limited vocabulary and often uses the same word to say several different things. He doesn't seem to understand the most elemental principles of language, that different things have different names. He says "Mommy" and "Daddy" but doesn't use many names, not even his own.

He has a cousin he really likes. Her name is Anna, and she's six years old. He says her name when he sees her, but he also calls his grandmother Anna. Anna and Lucas's grandmother live in the same house. It's a duplex, where Lucas's grandparents live in one part and their daughter and family live in the other. I wonder if that may be the reason they both get the tag "Anna." Does he associate the concept with the place and not the person?

I want to give him an understanding of language, that different things and people have different names. Lucas is very visually oriented. He loves to watch TV, and I latch on to that. I begin by teaching him the names of our closest relatives. Using the video camera, I film all the people in our surroundings while each one is saying his or her name. We record Lucas, and we say his name. Then we play the video on the TV. At first, he complains and doesn't want to watch, instead choosing some of his favorite movies, but I persist. Now we're going to watch. I hold him, and we sit on the floor in front of the TV and watch the video. We do that for a while every day. At the same time, during the day we point at different things and say their names.

Eventually, he begins to understand. Now he can point out people himself if we ask, for example, "Where's Sara?" When he has learned that, I continue and record various objects. Generalization can be difficult for autistic people. If, for example, they've learned that a specific ball is called "ball," then it can turn out that only that ball is called "ball," not any other ball of a different color or size. Therefore, I tape many balls of different colors and sizes.

Then we continue working with verbs, and Lucas slowly begins to understand language, something that other children do from an early age and pick up automatically. They totally absorb new words, like sponges. A one-year-old can't say much but has a huge passive vocabulary, an understanding of words that grows each day. When Lucas is three years old, he can barely speak and hardly has any passive vocabulary.

Parallel to the video, I work a lot with photographs. I take pictures of food, people, places, just about everything that has to do with Lucas's world. I soon realize that it's both expensive and time-consuming to develop photos, so I buy a digital camera, color printer, and a laminator, so we can laminate photos and they'll last longer.

At the computer resource center, Lucas is acquainted with the computer. We borrow computer programs to practice on. I find one on my own, The First Thousand Words, which is really for Swedes learning English but works just as well for learning Swedish.

An important foundation of communication is taking turns, something kids begin to learn at around six months of age. Taking turns is part of the BOEL test. The child is given a toy and asked to respond by giving it back, something Lucas couldn't do when he was eight months old. We visit the lekotek and borrow material that we use to play at communication and teamwork. We attach great importance to taking turns when we do play training. Playing is also a kind of dialogue. One child expects a reaction from the other child. If the reaction doesn't come, there won't be any play. Lucas loves to play tag, but when I've tagged him, he doesn't understand that it's his turn to chase me. I remember another time when Lucas stood and pulled a string through the back of a spindle-backed chair. A girl came and took the other end. It was obvious that she wanted to start a tug of war, but when she pulled the string, Lucas let go and walked away. He didn't understand that she expected a response or that he should pull his end. It is quite difficult to develop an interaction with someone who so totally lacks understanding of the concept.

Lucas can't speak, but that doesn't mean he doesn't have anything to say. He wants food, he's thirsty, he wants to play tag, and he wants to watch a certain movie. There is a lot he wants to say, but he doesn't know how. He uses some words, but mostly he points when he wants something. I want to help him communicate.

I find an inspirational book and buy a bulletin board, which I put up in the kitchen, our natural gathering place. I hang it on the wall, at the children's eye level. On it, I put photos of places we've visited, outings we've done, and people we know. Since Lucas doesn't speak, we can't talk about things, but we can gather around the pictures and share experiences. Together, we can point at the photos, and I can put words to our experiences.

The speech therapist had advised me to use signs to support Lucas's communication. After reading a lot about autism, I reevaluate that advice. Autistic people can have difficulties in abstract thinking, body awareness, and imitation. They can also have problems with memory. Signing is often abstract; it vanishes as soon as you've done it, and it can be hard to do if you have difficulty imitating and poor body awareness. Sign communication is also inherently limited, because it requires that the person you're communicating with understand the signs. Otherwise you can't communicate. Lucas is visual, and therefore I want to use pictures as an aid rather than signs.

I find an American method on the Internet, PECS (picture exchange communication system), that builds on a sender and a receiver. For Lucas, we make a little book of pictures of food, drink, and activities. There are also photos of different people he might like to meet. We teach him that he must give the picture to the person in order to get what he wants.

One Saturday, we go into town to do errands. Carl is driving, and Sara is in her car seat in the front. Lucas and I are in the back. On the way, we stop to get gas. The kids and I stay in the car and wait for Carl to finish. When he's done, he goes in to pay. Suddenly,

Lucas starts to point at his red picture book, which is on the seat next to me. I give it to him, and he turns the pages excitedly until he finds the right one. He shows me a picture that he puts next to a strip of paper with text that says, "I want . . ." and then gives me the whole sentence. I pick up the paper and read aloud, "I want some juice."

He looks at me. I feel warm all over. He can tell us what he wants!

"Would you like a juice?" I ask Lucas, and hold up the paper strip and photo so he can reach it. He points several times to the picture of the juice. I want to run in and tell Carl to buy a juice, but I can't get out of the car because the door locks are childproof. I find my cell phone and call him.

"Guess what? Lucas just 'PECSed' that he wants some juice," I say.

"That's great, but I just paid."

"Then you'll just have to go back in and get some. Buy one for Sara too. Get pear juice. They both like that."

Lucas's joy at being able to communicate is unmistakable when Carl comes back with juice for both of the kids.

Lucas learns the PECS system quickly. Most often, he tells us he wants to watch TV, play computer games, blow soap bubbles, drink juice, and eat cinnamon rolls. Sometimes, he tells us that he wants to eat sausage, without my asking him.

Carl and I don't often go out in the evening—the children are small, and it isn't easy for others to put them to bed and comfort them if they wake up at night. Sometimes, Carl and I go out separately, but then one or the other of us is at home. One evening, I'm out with friends and Carl is at home with the kids. They're all lying in our big double bed, Carl in the middle, with one child on either side. Sara has chosen a book, *Maisy the Mouse,* a fun kids' book with flaps that open. Lucas usually likes to lift the flaps to see what's on the other side. They lie and read, and Carl points to the pictures and talks. Suddenly, Lucas sits up and jumps off the bed. He runs out the door and down the hall.

"Lucas! Come back! We're going to bed now."

Carl hears Lucas go downstairs.

"Lucas! Come on! We're going to sleep!"

After a short while, he returns and climbs up into the bed and lies down next to Carl. He's holding the sentence strip of paper and a small picture that he hands to Carl. Carl reads, "I want Mommy."

He pulls Lucas close, hugs him, kisses his head, and breathes in his aroma before Lucas pulls free.

"I know, sweetheart. You miss Mommy. Mommy will be home later. She'll be here when you're asleep."

He's satisfied with the answer but insists on holding the picture in his hand as he falls asleep.

The same thing happens in the afternoon sometimes, when we're waiting for Carl to get home from work. Lucas gets out his paper strip, puts a picture of his dad on it, and gives it to me. He's longing for his dad.

ANOTHER WAY TO LEARN

It's been snowing for several days. A white blanket on the houses and gardens gives nature a magical feeling. The snow muffles all sharp sounds, but it crunches a little beneath my feet, and our sled grates when it hits a rock or a bare patch of pavement. I'm glad the snow has come early this year. Lucas loves the snow, and it's much easier for us to be outdoors then. We can wrestle in the snow and throw snowballs at the trees. He throws well for his age.

Sara is tucked into her carriage, asleep. Her sweet face is visible, and her cheeks are a faint red from the chill. Her snowsuit is checkered pink and white, and the fur lining of her hood is pulled tight around her head. She looks peaceful. I push the carriage and pull the little green sled. Lucas is on the sled; he drags his hand along the road, watching, fascinated as the snow piles up in his hand, then falls aside.

We walk on, and I gaze out over the bay. Ice has already formed on the water. It's been a cold December. We're on our way to the big meadow with the apple trees, where there's a good hill for sledding. All the kids in the neighborhood go there to ride their sleds and Snow Racers. Sometimes, you can see kids trying out their skis.

The meadow is often crowded on the weekends, but today there aren't very many kids on the hill. It's a weekday and most of them are in school. Some parents are at the top, chatting. I greet a couple of them I recognize and park the carriage a little farther away, so the parents' talking and the laughter and shouting of the children won't wake Sara.

At first, Lucas and I ride down the hill together. He's giddy with delight when we pick up speed. We have a good glide and end up almost at the apple trees. Some children are sledding next to us. They joke, overturn, and tumble around in the snow. They get up, excited, and run up the hill to do it again.

When the sled has stopped, I get out, but Lucas stays still.

"Come on, Lucas. Let's do it again."

He doesn't move, and I have to lift him out and put him on his feet. I take his hand, and we walk up the hill.

"Look at that girl," I say and point toward a little girl in a red snowsuit, who's coming down the hill at full speed. "See, when the sled stops, she gets up and walks back up the hill again. That's the way to do it."

Lucas doesn't look in her direction. He's busy kicking lumps of snow from his path. Next time, it's his turn to ride alone. He doesn't get as far this time, and stops far from the apple trees. Then he just sits there.

"Lucas, get up and come back up," I shout as loud as I can.

But he doesn't move. He just sits there.

"He seems to like it down there," a dad says to me, and laughs.

"He's just a little lazy," I reply, though I know it isn't true.

I run down the hill and lift him up from the sled.

"Do you want to do it again?"

He doesn't answer, but if he hadn't wanted to, he would have screamed no.

"Come on, let's walk up and have another ride."

He rides many times, and each time is the same. I have to run down and fetch him, and we walk back up the hill together.

A week later, I bring our video camera to the hill. I pretend I'm recording Lucas, but actually I zoom in on another little boy who's riding down the hill. I film how he rides down and, when the sled stops, how he gets up, takes the rope in hand, pulls the sled up the hill, and then rides down again. At home, I show Lucas the video on the TV. I point and tell him what the boy is doing.

The day after that, we return to the hill. It's early in the morning and we're the first ones there. Lucas rides down the hill by himself. Sara is awake and sits in the carriage, watching. The hill is fast, because it thawed and then froze again during the night. I'm afraid he'll ride too far, all the way to the trees, but the sled stops just in time. I hold my breath and wait. Did he understand what I tried to teach him?

For a while, Lucas just sits there, but then he gets up and begins to walk back up the hill, dragging the sled behind him. At the top, I wait, jumping up and down, clapping my hands above my head. Sara, in the carriage, starts clapping too.

"Good, Lucas!" I scream excitedly. "Great! Good work! Come, so you can ride again!"

The little figure comes toward me, smiling, and I'm filled with an indescribable joy.

Lucas lives in his own world. He doesn't observe people around him and doesn't imitate and learn that way. I know Lucas can learn, but he learns differently than normal children. I just have to find the right ways to help him.

DENIAL

I'm sitting at the kitchen counter, filling in a form. Lucas is watching TV, and Sara is pushing her doll carriage around. On Saturday, the psychologist is coming to begin testing Lucas for the assessment we're having done. Before the testing, we have to fill out a form, describing Lucas in as much detail as possible, from birth to the present. It contains both boxes to x in and open-ended questions. I write down everything that comes to mind. Carl reads it and makes additions. We want the psychologist to have as complete a picture of Lucas as possible.

A little later, my mother-in-law drops by. I tell her about the form and ask her to read what we've written to see if she wants to add anything. She sees Lucas often and knows him well. She reads silently, then erupts:

"But that's not Lucas at all! That's not right. How can you even express yourselves that way? This is *not* right! The psychologist will get the wrong impression of Lucas. I know that you think he's autistic," she says to me. "It shines through everything you've written here. It's as if you've copied it all from one of those books you've been reading."

I don't agree. We see Lucas in a very different light. She is blinded by her love of her grandchild. In her eyes, there's nothing wrong with Lucas. She means well, interprets the tiniest signal from him as communication and reads in what isn't there. She doesn't want to understand and can't accept the fact that he's different. There is nothing I would like better than for him to be normal, like other kids, but I can no longer just ignore reality. I want some kind of diagnosis. It doesn't matter if it's called autism or something else, as long as we can get help and support. With a heavy heart, I describe all his aberrant behaviors and failings. It destroys me to need to see him that way. Can't she understand that?

"I know we don't agree, but we've talked about it and we want you to write down your thoughts about Lucas and his development because you know him so well, so we can give that to the psychologist, too," I say. "That way, she'll get a more complete picture of him."

"I've already begun," she says.

For Carl and me, autism has a stigma. It feels abstract, scary, and awful. We didn't know much about it, and we have preconceived notions—that autistics are mentally retarded people who cannot speak, and sit and rock in a corner, doomed to live in their own isolated world. That was what we envisioned when we first heard the word "autism."

We'd noticed that the idea of autism slowly crept in and affected our way of seeing Lucas. The little boy we had three years ago wasn't the boy we thought he would be. It's as if we don't know him any-more. We have a new child. A child we see with new eyes, whom we believe requires completely different treatment. Suddenly, he isn't an ordinary little guy. He's odd, different, and we don't know how to act.

We begin searching for wrong and aberrant behaviors. We study what he does and how he reacts to various things. We see him in a new light.

Earlier in the fall, we went to Dubai for a week of vacation. We had flown together as a family many times before, but this time was different because now we thought Lucas might be autistic. How would it work? I was afraid he'd disturb other passengers on the plane. Naturally, he and Sara had disturbed people before—they're kids after all—but now I was extra careful that he wouldn't be a bother. I didn't want them thinking he was weird. I called and booked special seats, in the front by bulkhead with more leg room, a little more private, and Lucas would be able to sit on the floor or lie under a blanket, just like he loves to do sometimes when there's too much going on around him. Before the flight, I fretted a lot about how it would work out. Even my mother-in-law had some suggestions, despite the fact that she stubbornly maintained there was nothing wrong with him.

Before the trip, I made a small photo album of the steps we would go through. There was a picture of a taxi, since we would begin that way. After that, the airport, a check-in counter, the airplane taking off and landing, the baggage claim, the transfer shuttle, and finally the hotel and pool. Lucas loves to swim, and if he got restless during the trip, I could show him the pictures so he'd understand that at the end we'd reach the much longed-for destination.

The trip went fine, better than we expected, actually. On earlier flights, Lucas had screamed a lot and couldn't sit still. I don't know if it was the photo album that made the journey easier or if it was the fact that Lucas was older and more mature.

In Dubai, we stayed at a smaller hotel on a beach. There weren't many families there, which contributed to the feeling that all eyes were on us. We didn't want to disturb the other guests, so we were on extra good behavior. Sara was a little over a year old, and Lucas would soon be three. They had a lot of energy.

The first evening, we ate dinner in the hotel restaurant. Sara could sit in her child seat and was okay with what she had on her plate, but Lucas, who was very particular about what food he wanted, protested loudly when his hamburger looked different and smelled wrong. Luckily, the French fries were fine and he dipped them in ketchup, but as soon as he was finished, he wanted to leave. He refused to sit and wait, got up, and walked away. We had to run after him and haul him back to our table, with him wildly screaming in protest. I held him in my lap and tried to calm him, but to no avail. He screamed so much that he couldn't stay. We had to split up. I left with Lucas while Carl and Sara ate, then Carl came and relieved me, so I could finish my meal. After that, we ate at simpler restaurants or ordered room service.

There are fantastic shopping centers in Dubai, and that's where we went when we tired of the pool and the beach. They're huge, several stories high, and they often have food courts. In that noisy environment, it didn't matter that the kids didn't want to sit still and eat. There were playrooms where they loved to stay. There were rooms full of plastic balls to burrow in and exciting tunnels to crawl through. The escalators were another attraction for Lucas. He never tired of riding with us up and down between floors.

However, we spent most of our time at the beach or by the pool. We tried to get Lucas to build sand patties and castles, like his little sister, but he was mostly interested in standing and throwing sand into the water. Both of the kids liked the kiddy pool. Sometimes there were other kids there. Sara, young as she was, was immediately interested in them and tried to approach them, but not Lucas. I remember one boy trying to get Lucas's attention and make contact, but Lucas just ignored him and turned away. Lucas jumped around in the pool in a strange way, making strange noises. He spun around until he was completely dizzy and fell over. He behaved like a "retard," though he looked normal. It seemed to us that the other parents gave him weird looks, and we were ashamed of our son, our beloved little boy.

Our own feelings scared us, and we didn't want Lucas to have a label, an "autism" label. When people meet Lucas, they should form their own opinion of him rather than see him as an example of some diagnosis. We didn't want people to have preconceived notions that would affect how they acted and behaved with him, so we hid our suspicions from most outsiders. We kept them within the family. We didn't even mention them to my mother or my sisters. Only Carl's mom knew, because she was with us so often.

WHICH METHOD
SHOULD WE USE?

We understand that it's necessary for Lucas to practice in order to develop his communication and other skills. On weekdays, Carl's mom comes over and takes care of Sara while I work with Lucas, but it's hard to do everything in the time we have. Carl tells his childhood friend, Fredrik, about our dilemma. It turns out he's taken a leave-of-absence from his teaching job to write his thesis, and he offers to work extra with Lucas.

In mid-January, he starts working with Lucas. He comes over for a couple of hours each morning. We notice right away that Lucas is making progress. He no longer disappears into his own world, and he's interested in us and what's around him in a different way than he was before. Earlier, he only wanted to watch TV, but now he often comes and says he wants to "roll."

We've invented a game in our big bed. The bed is a good place to be, because it's a limited area and Lucas stays there and interacts. Otherwise, he can easily just disappear somewhere. We fold the blanket double, then Lucas lies on one end, and we roll him up in it. When he's completely rolled up, he's forced to say, "Roll!" before we roll him out again, fast. He loves to spin, and I believe the pressure from the blanket against his body feels good. Since he's motivated, we get him to say, "Roll."

His powers of concentration increase, and he can sit for long periods of time with Fredrik and practice different tasks, like taking turns building a tower of blocks or pointing out objects or people from pictures.

It's evening, and the children are asleep. Carl lies on the beige corner sofa in the living room and watches TV. I'm around the corner, in our smaller living room, called the music room. I sit curled up in the sofa, reading a thin yellow book, *Learning to Learn: An Approach to Language for Autistic Children*, by Gun-Louise Lyrén. I only get through a few pages when I call:

"Carl, I think I've found a method that suits Lucas!"

"That's nice," he says. "Which one is it this time? You're always finding new ones."

"Yes, but this one feels right."

I'm completely engrossed in the text. The book is easy to read, and I finish it in no time. Then I walk over to Carl and sit next to him on the couch.

"You need to listen to this." He reluctantly turns off the TV, and I begin to read aloud from the book.

Children learn something through some internal drive, a will to learn, but also because of various external rewards the child may receive, for example, praise, like an appreciative "Good work!" Children are motivated.

An autistic child lacks the internal drive and the ability to imagine something. The teacher must provide the drive, be the child's motor. An autistic child needs to learn motivation.

Children can remember and learn several parts of a task simultaneously. An autistic child must learn step-by-step and according to a certain structure.

Children learn a lot by imitating. That's how they learn language, everyday chores, games, and social interplay.

In order to learn to imitate, an autistic child must first learn to imitate on command.

Children learn something and can then apply it in different contexts and with different people. Children can generalize what they've learned.

An autistic child can't immediately generalize anything that's learned, but needs to learn to generalize.

For an autistic child, the way to learning goes via:

Motivation—structure—imitation—generalization.

"You see?" I say. "The method is based on the assumption that Lucas has a learning disability. He needs to 'learn to learn' before he can learn."

"Yeah, that sounds reasonable," says Carl.

"Believe it or not, this method is based on the Lovaas method," I explain.

"Wasn't that the one you thought was so terrible?" Carl asks.

"Well, yes, but *here* it seems sound. They use the Lovaas method as a model, but they adapt it for Sweden's way of life and value systems."

Ivar Lovaas was a Norwegian psychologist who worked with autistic children in the United States beginning in the 1960s, providing behavioral treatment that utilized the principles of applied behavior analysis. In the beginning, to do away with negative behavior in children, he used punishment in the form of electric shocks. I'd read many horrible articles about his method. ABA was once a rather brutal reward-and-punishment training program, but today's approaches are apparently very different.

I look up the author and call her. I tell her that I read her book and am interested in knowing more about this method. She's very helpful, describes it, and tells me there is a psychologist in Sweden who offers treatment and teaches courses in the method. The method goes by many names: CBT (cognitive behavioral therapy), ABA (applied behavior analysis), EIBI (early intensive behavioral intervention). She also gives me a tip on a group of parents with autistic children who are using this method. They're called the SITT (Swedish interest group for early intensive behavioral therapy).

I become even more convinced that this approach would suit Lucas, and I contact the psychologist, Örjan Swahn. He tells me that he was in the US in 1991, working at Professor Lovaas's clinic at UCLA, the world leader in the treatment of autism. When he returned to Sweden, he started his own clinic, where he gives counseling and consultation and teaches with an emphasis on behavioral disorders, communication training, and autism. I tell him that I'm scared by the electric shock treatments, but he answers that it's been a long time since they've been used. Today, physical punishment is no longer part of the treatment, at least not in Sweden, where the emphasis is instead on reinforcing positive behaviors.

Örjan tells me that a team is formed around the child, consisting of parents, a coach, and possibly preschool personnel. The training is very intensive, and the child practices with members of the team around thirty hours per week. It's a demanding process, so it's good to be able to shift between different trainers. Initially, it's mostly individual training with the child, but when the child develops the ability to interact, others are brought into it. Like, for example, adults known to the child, siblings, or friends. The exercises are tailored to the individual, and it's important to begin at the correct level in order to progress step by step. The child must always feel that he or she is succeeding, so that it's fun to learn. It's tough for the child at first, since he isn't used to this kind of intensive training, but the work is carried out in a pleasurable way and is constantly broken up by short recesses, so the child can relax and play freely.

When the child performs correctly, the trainer gives the child positive reinforcement; when the child errs, the trainer simply says, "Wrong." Since autistic children don't always appreciate praise, some other form of reinforcement may be needed, for example a piece of candy, a raisin, or something else that the child is fond of. In time, those reinforcements are abandoned and replaced with praise or a pat. The exercises are repeated many times, until the child knows them thoroughly. Exercises are generalized in many different ways and in different environments. Örjan says that most children don't have spoken language when they come to him, but many develop it after one or two years. All of his courses are booked up for the near future, but, since there is a large demand for them, he can plan an extra one. I think the method sounds good and I sign us up.

I contact one of the parents in the SITT group. She's very welcoming and describes the organization and how it works. I get the phone numbers of several parents, whom I call and speak with. They're all very helpful, giving advice and support. Their children were diagnosed several years earlier, while we are in the middle of it all now. I cry through some of the conversations, but all the parents give me fantastic support. They describe their own sorrow and tell me that it takes time before the first crisis is over, but assure me that, with time, you learn to handle and live with it all. It's hard to believe.

I learn a little more about how the training works and several of them praise the book, *Let Me Hear Your Voice* by Catherine Maurice, which they feel I should read. It's about an American woman who gives birth to an autistic child and how she tries several therapies to help her child. She interrupts several programs that do more harm than good, but, using intensive behavioral therapy, she succeeds in getting her child to start speaking, and, after a few years' training, her daughter has totally recovered. She had another baby, who is also autistic. The book describes how she repeats the treatment and how the second child is totally cured by the method. Both of her children were diagnosed with autism but after the training program, neither of them showed any autistic symptoms and they started school in normal classes.

The parents tell me that you can't count on your child being completely cured, but there is a chance. In the SITT group, one boy was, but he is the only one out of twenty children. He goes to a regular school, has no special aids, and doesn't need extra lessons. The other children have made great progress and might not have developed any language skills if it weren't for this therapy. This gives me hope for Lucas.

The parents tell me I can apply for support from the government and how much economic assistance we should demand and expect. In Sweden, if your child is diagnosed with autism, the child is covered by LSS—*Lagen om Stöd och Service till vissa funktionshindrade*, the Act Concerning Support and Service for People with Certain Functional Impairments—the law governing support and service for certain functionally challenged people. Yet, despite of the fact that there's a law, you're forced to fight tooth and nail to get what your child has every right to, they tell me. We're invited to come to the group's annual meeting on February 1.

THE EVALUATION

During December and January, they evaluate Lucas. We open our home to special needs teachers, speech therapists, and a psychologist, who come in turn to meet him and perform different tests. Lucas is being very good about it. There is no comparison to the testing with the speech therapist that we did in the fall, when he didn't want to participate and just ran around and threw toys. This time it's working out unbelievably better. For one set of tests, we were able to get Lucas to sit and stay concentrated for a whole hour. That took some bribing in the form of candy and short breaks for playtime, but he stuck with it for the hour.

During the psychologist's latest visit, she says she's seen Lucas make great progress during the past month. She wonders what we're doing, and I tell her about our training program. She says, "He's lucky to have parents like you."

I understand that she means well, but, I think, how can she even talk about luck when he has had the terrible bad luck to be born with a difficult handicap—not being able to communicate? He may never be able to speak, never be able to make himself understood. Maybe he'll always be dependent on others to interpret him and try to understand him and what he wants. I wouldn't want anyone to become so fettered and "un-free," and *she* talks about luck.

A couple of months later, after the psychologist's tests have been completed, Carl and I meet with Tore Duvner. We talk about Lucas, and he asks us questions. At the next appointment, he meets with Lucas.

It's cold outside, and there is still a lot of snow. We take the car and drive the short distance in a few minutes. It's hard to imagine that he's so close! Lucas jumps out of the car and picks up pieces of snow, throwing them at me.

"Calm down, Lucas," I say. "Come on, we're going into this building to visit a nice man who lives here."

I take his hand, and we climb the stairs to the building. The brick edifice is up on a small knoll. It's early afternoon and quiet in the neighborhood. Carl rings the doorbell, and it's Duvner who opens the door. He has kind eyes and is approaching seventy. You can tell he's used to meeting people with great burdens of sorrow. I feel he has a special kind of respect. I almost want to cry when I see him.

"Hello and welcome," he says.

His face lights up when he says hi to Lucas. I feel he must be a great children's doctor. We enter the hall and take off our coats. As usual, Lucas kicks off his boots and pulls off his socks. Then he's gone. Instead of entering the reception area on the ground floor, he has run up the stairs into Duvner's private quarters.

Duvner laughs.

"I'll go up and get him," he says. "Come on in." He waves a hand in toward the examination room, but we stay out in the hall. It takes a while before they come down again.

"He found an exciting closet up there," he says and smiles at us. "Come on, Lucas, we're going in here instead. There're fun things in here too."

We enter his office, consisting of two rooms. The interior decoration looks like it's from the 1960s. In the first room, there's a mustard-colored sofa by one wall and a large, soft, rectangular rug in front of it. Large windows open out toward the back garden. In one corner of the garden, I see a swing swaying lightly in the breeze.

Carl and I sit on the sofa, and Lucas crawls into my lap. Duvner sits in an armchair across from us. We begin to talk. Duvner wants Lucas to feel safe before he does any observation of him. After a while, Lucas gets up and walks around the room, beginning to

examine things. There are many different toys on a shelf in the corner next to the sofa.

After a while, Duvner asks me and Carl to go into the other
room. The door is open and Lucas can see us the whole time. Duvner
stays with Lucas and approaches him by showing interest in the toys
Lucas chooses. He tries to get him to play and interact. Suddenly,
Lucas runs in to us, but then he returns to Duvner. He seems to be
comfortable with him, and Duvner keeps him busy for a long time.
Meanwhile, Carl and I sit in the room next door and try to make
ourselves uninteresting. After a while, I see from the corner of my
eye that Lucas is beginning to feel the need to go to the bathroom.

I follow him to the toilet out in the hall. When he's finished, he
washes his hands. He plays with the running water. I try to get him
to come back, but he refuses. Duvner hears that he won't come. He
calls to me that it doesn't matter. He thinks he's seen enough. I leave
Lucas in the bathroom and return. Carl and I sit in the sofa again,
and Duvner sits across from us.

He tells us what he's seen in his time with Lucas, noting interaction,
eye contact, and communication. He thinks Lucas shows signs of a serious speech and communication disorder and has a few autistic traits.
He can't give us a diagnosis now, without first going over the tests that
the speech therapist and psychologist have done. We get a new appointment for February 7, to meet and receive the diagnosis. I can feel tears
coming on. Carl squeezes my hand. I look at him and see that his eyes
are reddish. Duvner gives me a Kleenex from a box he has nearby. The
discreet, small boxes are in many places in both rooms. I wonder how
many parents have sat here and felt sorrow over their child, who won't
get to live a normal life like other children. I blow my nose and dry
my tears. Lucas is still running the water in the sink, so I go into the
hall again. When I open the bathroom door, the sink is full of white
froth bubbling over the edge and running onto the floor and the green
bathroom rug. The soap pump next to the faucet appears empty. Lucas
doesn't turn around; he's busy with the lather and looks very focused.

SEVEN DAYS IN
FEBRUARY

It's early February. This week, a lot is happening. On Saturday, Carl and I have been invited to the yearly meeting of SITT (Swedish interest group for early intensive behavioral therapy). All the members train their kids using behavioral therapy. It'll be exciting to meet other parents and learn some of their experiences. The meeting takes place at one of the parents' homes. They live in a turn-of-the-century building right on the St. Eriksplan plaza, in a chic and very upscale part of Stockholm. We ring the bell, and a woman opens the door. We step into their newly renovated apartment, which is very tastefully decorated. She asks if we'd like an espresso, cappuccino, latte, or macchiato. We follow her into the modern kitchen, where we're served coffee. Several parents stand talking around the island in the middle. We're introduced to some new parents, who are beginning behavioral therapy. Everyone welcomes us and thinks we've made the right decision about Lucas's training. This method is the only one that has the research to prove it helps autistic children develop. Many of the parents combine behavior therapy with diets and supplements to stimulate the brain. We're struck by how knowledgeable and driven the parents seem to be.

We get to meet the father of the boy who has been completely cured and who goes to a regular school. The other children receive different kinds of special education and, according to their parents, have made enormous progress. At the meeting, we're talking to a mom, Lotta, and tell her that we have a tutor for Lucas but that he has only another couple of months left. Lotta says that she has done the training herself with her son and will be looking for work, now that her youngest is going to begin at preschool. She's a nurse but wants to do something new. She offers to start training Lucas.

What luck! Everyone has mentioned how hard it is to find competent trainers who know the method. Here we get the opportunity to have an experienced trainer who is also a parent, and who knows what it's like to have a child that's different. We decide to have Lotta come visit and meet Lucas the following week, to get to know him and talk more about how we might continue. This happy prospect gives us hope for a treatment that will work.

Early in the week, we go to Uppsala to take part in a course in behavioral therapy given by Örjan Swahn, the psychologist who had explained the method to me. Just as Örjan had asked, we have with us a team of people from Lucas's immediate circle. They won't all be training him, but as Örjan explained, this method is all about a perspective that permeates everything you do, and it's good if as many people as possible in Lucas's environment can learn the method, to be able to help him develop. They comprise Grandmother and Grandfather, my in-laws; my mother and her husband, Ingvar; Vera, a teacher at the preschool Lucas will be attending; Fredrik, Carl's childhood friend who helps with Lucas's training; and Lotta, the parent from SITT who will also train Lucas. And then there are Carl and myself, and of course Lucas, the main character.

The course will last for two whole days. We have brought Lucas's favorite toys: a spinning top, a flashlight, and bubble soap. We've also brought chocolate, potato chips, and Coca Cola. All of these things will be used as reinforcement in the training, that is, our rewards for Lucas when he succeeds with various tasks. We also have the video camera, to be able to record everything if we want to go back later and watch what we did and even to be able to show the relatives how the training works.

Örjan Swahn receives us at his study center, a simple, low brick building. As we enter, there is a long corridor, broken up by several doors along the sides leading into treatment rooms. We total four families, and it's a large group of people, with all the relatives and tutors who've come along. First, we all gather, and Örjan tells us about the method and about what will happen in these two days. Then each family gets its own room to work in. We rig the video camera and get going.

The first thing Lucas will learn is to listen and understand the command "Come here." He has never come when we've called him before, but now he'll learn how to do it. I sit on a low children's stool, three feet in front of Lucas. Örjan stands behind him and holds him. Then I call.

"Lucas! Come here!"

When I call, Örjan "prompts" him. That means he helps him a little by pushing him in my direction. When Lucas comes to me, I hug him, and everyone in the room claps and exclaims, "Good, Lucas!"

Lucas is embarrassed at first, but eventually I see how he begins to appreciate the praise, and he looks around to get everyone's praise when he has performed correctly. We repeat it again and again. If Lucas doesn't move, Örjan says, "Wrong," I call again, and if he doesn't come on his own Örjan helps him with a push toward me. When he gets it right spontaneously, he receives a little piece of potato chip as a reward. Once he can run to me, we trade off and other people call for Lucas. Finally, several people sit in a circle and take turns calling him, and he runs from person to person.

Örjan has explained that there are a few basic skills Lucas needs to master to be able to begin with more difficult tasks. Lucas must be able to come when called, he must be able to sit still on a chair, and he must be able to maintain eye contact with the person who's training him. These things are the first we work on, and it takes time. Lucas doesn't want to have eye contact. Örjan has to hold up a piece of potato chip between his own eyes in order to get Lucas to look at him. When Lucas gives eye contact, he gets the potato chip and we clap and tell him how clever he is. It's just as important for us to learn how to work with Lucas as it is for him to learn these things. We must be extremely clear and use short instructions, with no unnecessary talk that may confuse Lucas. We are to reward him when he performs correctly, so he learns what he must do, and to say "wrong" when we don't get the desired response.

Lucas is clever, and we do many different things. He learns to sort similar things. We lay out two plastic plates on the table, one yellow and one pink. Then we give Lucas a pink plate and say, "Find the same one," and then Lucas is supposed to lay his pink plate on top of the pink one. He learns to do that fast. Then he learns to imitate us. There are two blocks on the table. I say, "Do this," and throw one of the blocks into a box on the floor. Lucas learns quickly to do the same.

We build with Lego blocks. Lucas and I sit across from each other at a table. In the middle is a flat red Lego base to build on. In front of me, I have put together a yellow and a green block to form a line. I have done the same in front of Lucas. Then I take a red block, say, "Do the same," and put it on top of my yellow block. I give Lucas a red block, and he's supposed to build identically with his blocks. When he succeeds, we vary the patterns that we build and make it more difficult. The exercise helps him learn to observe and imitate.

After that, we practice something that's called imitation. Örjan sits on a little child's stool across from Lucas. He says, "Do this," and claps his hands once. Lucas sits, turning and twisting on his stool, but he doesn't clap his hands. He picks his nose and then sneezes, so the snot runs down his face. Grandmother is quick to come and clean his face, but Örjan doesn't want us to give him any attention, since that is Lucas's way of avoiding the training.

During the previous training sessions, we all clapped our hands when Lucas succeeded with the exercises, and then he also clapped spontaneously, but now, when he's supposed to imitate, he can't. The next time Örjan claps, an assistant is standing behind Lucas, and when Lucas doesn't clap, the assistant puts Lucas's hands together as if to clap. Lucas screams and protests. Then Örjan claps again, and, instead of clapping, Lucas tries to give Örjan a slap. He cries, screams, sneezes, struggles, and tries to run away.

We all feel a little down at heart. The other exercises have gone well, with some protests from Lucas, but not like this. Örjan thinks it's good that Lucas reacts like this here and now, rather than when we're at home.

"You see here an example of an exercise that Lucas thinks is difficult. He becomes frustrated and doesn't want to participate any longer. It's possible he feels the expectation that he must perform and, when he can't do it, he just wants to flee," says Örjan. He continues, "Have we talked about moving out?"

"No," we answer.

"When you're moving out, there's always something that's extra fragile. It could be Grandma's heirloom crystal or the expensive stereo that you've packed in a box, and often it's precisely that box, which is supposed to be handled carefully, that you drop on the floor. It can be similar for Lucas. He wants to get it right, but if the exercise is difficult for him, he may freeze up and fail instead."

"What do we do if that happens?" I ask.

"It will happen repeatedly," says Örjan. "We know that. As it stands now, we could say that Lucas has too much will and too little understanding. We need to prescribe the treatment, because he wouldn't choose what's best for him. We know that children who go through this training make progress and develop their intellect. It's immensely important that the training be done in the right way, so we don't pressure him too much. He must feel that he can succeed at the exercises, and it's important to not go too fast and not too early into the exercises that he feels are difficult."

There is a long discussion about how we should relate to the training and how we'll be able to create a balance so that Lucas will feel good and comfortable with the training. When we drive home, we're filled with new impressions. It feels good, because we finally have a structured method to work with. We'll receive consistent coaching from Örjan about how to work and suggestions for new exercises as Lucas develops.

On Wednesday, the day after the course, we have an appointment with Duvner. We drive in silence along the familiar road. We have lived so long not knowing, but now we'll finally have an answer, we'll get the diagnosis. We are composed and prepared for the worst. He asks us to come into the back room. We seat ourselves in armchairs with Duvner across from us. He begins to explain what he interprets from the tests and then summarizes:

"Lucas is a boy with great difficulties in communicating. He has clear deficiencies in contact, interplay, and communication behaviors but still shows, in observation of play behavior and test situations, an interest in the various adults conducting the tests and certain imitation skills as well as interest in simple interplay. He has a controlled and careful way of playing and making physical contact and accepts verbal limitations. His gross and hand motor abilities are well-developed." Duvner thinks his collection of symptoms coincides with an autism spectrum disorder.

In spite of the fact that it's not a surprise, it hurts to hear it. My heart aches. Carl and I hold each other's hands, and both of us cry.

Duvner also finds that Lucas has normal intelligence and that he has a speech impediment. He says that, taking into consideration his speech disorder and that he shows as much interest as he does in contact and has quickly learned to communicate with pictures, one may hope that his autistic symptoms are secondary to his speech impediment. When we hear this, a little light is lit in the darkness.

The next day, Lucas and I are scheduled to visit the Lidingö Home preschool. I've already been there once to check it out and was impressed, the personnel were all so considerate and the activities so well organized and carefully prepared. The preschool is located in a large, comfortable house with a lovely garden. They want to meet Lucas and do a developmental evaluation to see if he can fit in.

We've already decided to start with behavioral therapy, and Lucas has received a place next fall at the Montessori preschool his cousins attend. While we're not really very interested in a spot at the Lidingö Home for the moment, I still want to keep all doors open. You never know what can happen and, besides, it's always good to get a second opinion.

A speech therapist greets us. First, we spend a while in the playroom, and Lucas runs around and looks at all the toys and other things there. The speech therapist takes Lucas upstairs. At first, he doesn't want to go, so I come along. After a while I can return downstairs, sit in the kitchen, and have a cup of coffee while the test is under way. I wonder how it's going. Will she also say that he seems to be autistic? After forty-five minutes, they come downstairs.

"How'd it go?" I ask.

"Lucas did great. It's obvious he's used to sitting down and training. We were able to complete a lot of the exercises. He didn't do some because he didn't understand the verbal instructions."

"No," I say. "Language is his biggest problem."

"Yes, but I also think he has some deficiency in his interplay, and he avoids eye contact."

"Yes, of course. What do you think, then? Is there any possibility he can start here?"

"Not from the way it looks today. He's still too young to benefit from our activities, but he could develop more during the spring. If his development speeds up, then it would be different. I think we should get back in touch before summer, and if you're still interested, we can do a new evaluation."

"Okay," I say, "that sounds good."

"You have a charming little boy," she says.

Then she tells me something she thought was remarkable. She asked Lucas to draw something on a piece of paper. He began to make a lot of dots on the paper, and then he drew lines connecting the dots. The lines became a house.

I smile, because I understand exactly why he did that.

LOVE IS NOT ENOUGH

When the speech therapist from Duvner's assessment team had been at our place, she noticed that Lucas couldn't draw. He did what small children do and tapped the pencil on the paper, making dots. She showed us a way to teach Lucas systematically to build up a drawing, by us first putting the dots on a paper and then teaching him to connect them with a line. In that way, he could learn to draw a house, a boat, a car, or any other object. We'd done this, but now Lucas had taken it one step further. Since there were no dots on the paper, he began by making them, and then he finished the drawing.

This Sunday, it will be ten years since my father died. My mom, my sister, our kids, and I will visit the grave. My youngest sister, Charlotta, is married. They had kids first and now have two children who are a year older than mine. My middle sister, Eva, is single and has no kids. Eva comes with us, and my mom rides with Charlotta. We talk about Dad.

The same memories pop up each time I think of him. Maybe we're at an airport, maybe we're somewhere else. My eyes seek him in the sea of people and find him standing, tall and handsome, a little to the side of all the people. He sees me, waves, and I run toward his outstretched arms. He bends down to meet me. Often tanned, with sun-bleached wisps in his brown hair, nonchalantly combed to the side. His blue eyes shine, and his mouth is one big smile, his white teeth against his dark beard. I can see his huge embrace, with his long arms outstretched.

"Hey, sweetheart! How big you've gotten," he says when he closes me in a bear hug, and his beard tickles my cheek.

For a moment, it's just the two of us. I have no idea where my sisters are, for it's just us, but they are surely there too. I don't remember any goodbyes, just our hellos. Now he's gone, gone forever. He died in a car crash ten years ago, before I had my twenty-fourth birthday.

Mother and Father divorced when I was around eight years old. Before that, we lived in Norrtälje and then in Portugal for a few years, for Dad's job. He designed clothing that he sold in Scandinavia.

After the divorce, we moved to a small town in Småland, where Mom's siblings and parents lived. We saw Dad on school holidays. We always felt a little different, having a Stockholm accent and a father who was never at home. Our budget was tight. Mother was a teacher with three kids to support. Money for everyday life, clothes, shoes, and things that growing children need was not something our father understood, and he was sporadic in paying child support. He saw it as his duty to teach us about life and the world outside the forests of Småland. On vacations, we often traveled. Buyers' trips to Paris, vacations in Rome, camel rides in Africa, sailing in Greece and the former Yugoslavia. It was exciting to experience exotic places, and we had a lot to tell our schoolmates. So it didn't matter that I never got that bike I wished for, because I got something that no one else had experienced.

On summer vacations, we stayed with Mother in the house in Portugal, which was still ours. When we were older, Father encouraged us to travel on our own. It was his idea that we should go to the US as exchange students. We received around-the-world airline tickets from Dad when we graduated from high school. I spent a year and a half traveling the world with my sister, Eva. We worked in bars and restaurants. I was also a nanny in France and studied Spanish in Mexico. When my dad was in his forties, he sold his company, bought a thirty-foot sailboat, and sailed around the world. I came along for six months on a trip from Rio de Janeiro, up through the West Indies to the US. I believe he lived his life the way he wanted to, but I regret that he isn't alive. He never met Carl or our children. He died much too early.

We arrive at the cemetery. The church is beautiful, majestically placed on a hill. It's a peaceful, early morning, and we're alone there. We decorate the grave. Cut away dead branches from the little juniper and light candles. The kids run around and play tag. Charlotta says that they should calm down. In a cemetery, you should show respect. There's no one else there, and I feel they can play if they want to. Dad wouldn't have minded, I'm sure.

Afterwards, I drive the kids home myself. The others ride together to visit some friends in Norrtälje. I don't feel like it, because I'm overcome with sorrow and just want to be alone with my tears and my kids. I remember what it was like ten years ago when Dad died.

I was at Stockholm University, living in student housing. On a Saturday evening, I got home late after my part-time waitressing job.

It's quiet on our corridor. I unlock my door, and the first thing I see when I enter the dark room is a blinking red light on my answering machine. I press the button, and first I hear the wind, then my dad's familiar voice.

"Jenny, sweetheart. This is your dad calling from Skåne. I've just been visiting with an old and dear friend down here. I'll probably be in Stockholm on Wednesday or Thursday. It's so cold down here in Simrishamn. I'm down at the harbor, and it's windy and snowing and colder than the bejeezus! Okay, have a good one, sweetie pie. See you later! Bye now!"

The sound of his voice makes me glad. It's been a long time since I've seen him, but next week I'll see him again.

On Sunday morning, I wake up at dawn. I wonder what woke me up and lie in bed, listening, but it's very quiet. I feel so awake, even though I fell asleep only a few hours ago. It takes a while before I manage to drop off again, but then I sleep a deep and long sleep.

Later, that evening, Mom calls. Her voice sounds strange.

"What's wrong?" I ask her. She doesn't reply.

"Come home for dinner," she says.

"It's late, and I need to study," I reply. I don't feel like getting on the subway and making the long trip out to Rågsved.

"Eva's on her way. Please come. I want to see you."

Her voice is brittle, and it scares me.

"What's wrong? Tell me!"

"Just get here as fast as you can. We can talk then." Her voice breaks and she hangs up.

I understand that it's serious and hurry out. I get on the subway and go there.

I walk the short stretch from the underground to the apartment complex. When I ring the doorbell to the apartment, Mother opens the door, the door and I can see at once that something's happened. Her face is grayish and empty. Mother hugs me and starts crying.

"What *is* it?" I ask.

"There's been an accident. Your dad may be dead," she sobs.

"Dead? How? He was coming here this week."

"The police called a while ago. They think he crashed the car this morning on the way up to Stockholm."

"They *think*? Don't they know?"

"They found a crashed car this morning with a deceased driver. The car had burned up, and they were unable to identify the body. They couldn't even read the license plate."

"How do they know it's Dad?"

"The police had the car towed and examined it. They found a chassis number and succeeded in tracking it to a car rental agency. It was your father who'd rented the car."

"But maybe it wasn't Dad who was driving?" And I hear how unreasonable it sounds. Who would be driving otherwise? He was on his way up to us for a visit.

"I believe we must prepare ourselves for the worst," says Mom.

"But how could he crash?" I say through my tears. "He's such a good driver."

"The police who called said there was low visibility and black ice on the road. It was snowing heavily. They think his car skidded. He crashed into a tree, and the car must have caught fire. An early morning snowplow discovered it, but by then the car was engulfed in flame. The driver couldn't do anything to help."

We sit the whole evening and hold each other, crying. We wait to call Charlotta, who lives in Argentina. We don't want her to be alone when she gets the message. On Monday, we read in the paper:

Driver dies in burning vehicle
One person died on Sunday morning in a single-car crash,
on Highway 35 in northern Kalmar County.
The car veered off the road and hit a tree. It ignited and
was completely burned when the police arrived at the scene.
At the time, it was dark, and there was snowfall. The road
was covered in thick ice.

It can't be true. He can't just be gone. Maybe it wasn't him in the car. Maybe it's all a hoax. I get out my old school atlas and look at the map. I want to know where he died, where the place is located, where he veered off the road and crashed the car. I find the lake. Not far from there is a village called Jenny.

We live in uncertainty for a few days. Was it Dad in the car, or was it someone else who died in the flames? After a week, we receive the news. They've examined his dental records, and they coincide with the deceased person. There is no doubt about it. Our father died in the accident.

Tearfully, I drive home from Norrtälje toward Stockholm again. It all comes back, as if it happened yesterday, but I need to be strong, especially for my kids. Old sorrows and new ones—I'm getting used to driving around in my car and weeping. But a mom who does nothing but cry isn't a good mother, and I bite the bullet, turn up the car radio, and force life to go on.

The diagnosis puts us in contact with a new world. We now have it in black and white that ours is a special needs child, one that demands more care than other children, and one that costs more.

In the fall, Lucas will be starting preschool. He will then be over three and a half years old. During the spring, the preschool assists us in applying for funding for a one-on-one paraprofessional for Lucas. We want the decision to be made and done before the summer, so that the preschool has time to find someone good, someone who can stay at Lucas's side and help him develop.

Earlier, before we got the diagnosis, I joined the Autism Society. I've read their information and gone to some courses but haven't participated in any of their activities. Now that we have a diagnosis, I feel the need to meet other parents in similar situations, and I'm curious about what their children are like.

The Autism Society arranges a meeting for parents and their recently diagnosed children at a special facility called the Lagoon, which offers specialized activities for people who are functionally challenged. It has six experiential rooms, each with its own theme. The environment is sensorially stimulating and can encourage either activity or relaxation. In the music room, you can listen to music and sounds or create them. On the waterbed there, the experience feels extra strong, since the sound vibrations pass through your whole body. There are many instruments to try out, the big wooden drum, the guitar, or the South American rainsticks. In the white room, there is a heated water bed along with many light effects—lava lamps, a mirror ball that slowly spins, fiber optics that shimmer. The music affects the mood in the room. Visitors can choose different light effects by pressing a button. In the darkened room, there are objects to touch and examine, luminous bugs, a vibrating snake, a shining ball. You can also move to music in the light of a mirror ball or feel the pulse in a vibrating beanbag chair. The room's design facilitates focusing on one thing at a time. The visitor can steer the various effects by means of a slight pressure on a button. In the boat room, where a boat is suspended from the ceiling and swings to the sound of lapping waves, surrounded by gulls, fishnets, and a small dock, you can pretend to cast off, taking along a fishing pole or a ship's cat, and feel the breeze. In the ball room, even those with physical handicaps can experience movement. Primarily balance, touch, and joint and muscle senses are stimulated in the ball room. Among other things, there is a trampoline, a swing, and various kinds of balls, large, small, spiny, and knobby, that you can play with or just feel. There is also a giant ball pool.

Five families are visiting the Lagoon. In order to limit the number of children, siblings are not allowed to come. There are three boys there, besides Lucas, and one girl. Some researchers have shown that three out of four children with a diagnosis within the autism spectrum are boys; others maintain it is as many as four out of five.

The kids are excited and are everywhere. They run between the rooms and discover new things. You can tell that they have similar social deficits because they barely seem to notice to each other.

I talk with the other parents. They are all more or less in a state of shock. Most of them had understood that something was different about their child, but didn't realize that they were autistic. One mother tells me that, at birth, she noticed her child was different. She believed he was mentally retarded, but the doctors didn't take her anxiety seriously and it took until he was almost three years old before he received a diagnosis. She tells me that she always has to keep an eye on him. I see him rushing around and notice as he puts his hand in a pot, takes some soil, and stuffs it in his mouth. He doesn't speak, just makes sounds. None of the children are talking, even though they're between three and five years old. A couple of them use a few single words. I study the other kids on the sly. Several of them are still in diapers. Somehow, it's comforting to see that others are having a hard time, just like us. Sometimes, when my life feels unbearable, I think of those who have an even heavier burden, and mine doesn't feel that bad. If others are strong and can get through things, then of course we can too.

HAVE WE CHOSEN THE RIGHT METHOD?

Lucas's training continues. Lotta works with him one morning a week, and Fredrik has the other weekdays. On the weekend, I work with Lucas. The exercises are going well, and Lucas is making progress. He seems to have had a breakthrough, for he can imitate clapping hands and we've continued on to other body imitation, like stamping your feet, patting your tummy, and jumping up and down on both feet.

He doesn't say much. He has a handful of words that he uses. His passive vocabulary is growing very fast, however. We lay out pictures, and he points out different objects. He learns new words quickly and points to the correct images. Lotta thinks he's ready for verbal imitation, that is, sound exercises. We agree to try it at the next counseling session with Örjan.

An exercise that, in spite of lots of practice, doesn't go well is learning colors. Lucas is supposed to learn to name all the colors. We've decided to begin with red. We lay down a red block and a plastic cow on the tabletop. Then we say, "Give me red," and Lucas is supposed to give us the red block. We prompt him—help him to choose the right one repeatedly, but when he has to do it himself, he most often chooses the cow. He truly doesn't understand. Maybe he's confused? After learning that a block is called a block, suddenly the block is red, something very different. Outside of training time I try to explain and show him that different objects have different colors. I talk about the clothes he wears, toys he likes, and many other things that are around us, but the concept of color seems to be beyond him.

Fredrik thinks it may help his learning if Lucas works with something he likes. Lucas loves M&M's, and we've used them as reinforcers, rewards, when he succeeds with the exercises. Now Fredrik begins to use M&M's in the exercises. He lays out one green and one red M&M on the table and says, "Point to red." If Lucas points correctly, he gets to eat the candy. If he points wrong, he doesn't, and they start over. For my part, I'm not sure that will make it any easier, and I believe Lucas is still pointing wrong about half the time, but Fredrik says that he's learning better now, since he's more motivated. When I try the same exercise, Lucas points wrong about half the time.

My father-in-law took the course in ABA with us, and he knows that it's based on Lovaas's methods. He gives me a tip, that I should visit the website amazon.com and read reviews of Lovaas's book, *Teaching Developmentally Disabled Children: The Me Book.* I read many reviews that praise the method and describe what an enormous help it's been in their child's development. Then I read a review that is diametrically opposed. It maintains that the method is too brutal and that children can develop post-traumatic stress syndrome from it. Instead, the reviewer recommends a method called "incidental teaching," which is based on the child's interests and builds on shared control and functional communication. The starting point is the child's own initiative to make contact, which would give a more lasting result.

I begin to worry that we've chosen the wrong method. The training has gone well, without a lot of protest, but I think I see Lucas showing some signs of stress. For a while now, he has had tics. At the moment, that entails him walking around and blowing his nose straight out into the air. I think this has increased, and now he walks around snorting most of the time. It doesn't look nice, because he blows and blows until he has a long string of snot hanging from his nose, and he wipes it off with his sleeve. Lucas has been free of diapers for a long time, but he has begun to wet and mess his pants again. We began potty training early with Lucas, and when he was two and a half he was diaper-free. He learned quickly, and it was unusual for him to wet his pants, but now he does it several times a day. I suspect it could be a sign of stress. Lucas can't say how he feels, and maybe this is a way for him to show it.

After a couple of weeks of ABA behavior therapy, we drive back to Uppsala for counseling.

We go through the exercises Lucas has done and explain that colors have been difficult. Örjan tries it with Lucas, but Lucas doesn't point out the red block. Fredrik, who feels that he succeeds better with M&M's, want to show Örjan, but that doesn't work well either.

Örjan says that color is an abstract concept and can be very difficult to understand. He thinks we should try another approach. When we say, "Red" now, Lucas doesn't seem to listen and appears to point haphazardly at the objects lying on the table. Örjan wants Lucas to listen more attentively. Immediately upon the request "Point to red," he wants him to have made a decision about which object he will point to. To accomplish this, he pulls Lucas's chair back from the table. Lucas is now seated a yard away from it. Örjan starts with an exercise Lucas knows. He puts a cow and a car on the table and instructs Lucas that he is to walk immediately to the side of the table where the selected object lies. In this way, Örjan believes Lucas will listen better to what we're saying, and this will lessen his impulsivity. Before he chooses an object, he must first decide which one he wants, so he can walk to the correct side. He suggests that we should try this at home with the concept "red" and see if it works better.

Lotta mentions that she would like to start with verbal imitation because she thinks Lucas seems ready for it. So Örjan does some test exercises with Lucas. He sits on a child's chair facing Lucas, so close their knees are almost touching. Örjan says, "Say, 'Bah,'" and Lucas imitates him and says the same thing. When Örjan tries a few different combinations, Lucas succeeds with some, but not all. Örjan has emphasized that you should never say, "Wrong," when Lucas fails to imitate and instead should say, "Nice try," or nothing at all. We are not to make any demands on his performance in speaking, and every sound he makes must be positively responded to, even if he doesn't succeed in imitating. If the sound is too difficult, we must quickly change to something that Lucas can say, for example "Mom" or "Dad," and then round off the exercise when Lucas feels he has succeeded. Örjan thinks we should start with nonsense words, which lessens the pressure to perform.

I wonder what Örjan thinks of incidental teaching and tell him I've read about it on the Internet. Örjan replies that he thinks it's good, but the method is slow. Since autistic children have difficulties communicating, there are not enough chances during the day to teach Lucas to communicate. Autistic kids are often independent and don't come asking for help. They don't usually play with other kids, and therefore there are few natural chances to learn. Behavior therapy is more effective, and the more Lucas learns, the more we can use incidental teaching in everyday life. I'm satisfied with his answer.

I also wonder what will happen to Lucas's self-esteem if we always decide what he must do. What can we do to reinforce his self-esteem and how shall we get him to develop better self-awareness? Örjan says that's what we're working on and that it comes automatically with the training. The more Lucas learns, the more he'll understand his surroundings, and he can take up more space and make himself understood better.

I bring up the fact that he's peeing his pants, and Örjan says that, in the beginning, that can happen, since the adjustment for the child is an effort, but it will pass.

We're working with behavioral therapy, but I also want to learn other methods. Anything that can facilitate Lucas's communication is good. I take a course in how to use digital pictures as an aid in communication and another in how you can make your own computer programs, tailored to your child. I make a picture presentation that is about Lucas, with images of him, what he likes to do, the food he likes. Pictures of his family, the house, and the preschool he'll go to. All to strengthen his sense of self and get him to understand that he is part of a context. At first, he won't look at the picture show, but then he gets used to it and starts to point to the people he sees on the screen and the things he does.

Lucas still has difficulty understanding the concept of color. Trying to make it clearer for him, I create a slide show with photos and sounds, using pictures of various red objects. The show begins with a red screen and my voice saying, "Red." The next picture is of a red car: you see the image and hear "Red car." The show consists of a number of different objects. Lucas and I sit together at the computer and take turns choosing different pictures. My hope is that he'll develop a feeling of what color is from doing this repeatedly. After red, I'm going to move on to other colors.

To prepare Lucas for the preschool he'll attend, I visit the school and take photographs of the kids, the personnel, the classrooms, and the playground. Then I put together a slide show about a day at preschool. It starts with a picture of Lucas, so he'll understand that he is the one who's going to preschool. After that, pictures of everything they do there in order, from opening the door and walking in, taking off his coat and putting it on its own hook, taking off his shoes, meeting, training, playtime, lunch and, when he's done, how to carry his plate from the table and scrape off the leftovers, going to the lavatory, and finally being outside in the yard. The last pictures are of me coming to pick Lucas up and then our house, so he'll understand that we go home. I want him to know how his day will look. It's hard to explain using only words, but with pictures, I think it's clearer to him.

At the computer course, I meet other parents who have kids with various handicaps. I'm the only one who has an autistic child, but one of the course administrators tells me that she has a grown son who is autistic. I wonder how things have gone for him and if he has learned to talk.

"No," she says. "He doesn't speak and can't tell us what he wants, but when I call at the group home to say hi and he hears that it's me, he starts singing lullabies he learned by heart."

It breaks my heart. I wonder if he would have been able to learn to speak if he had received some other kind of training. Previously, autistic children weren't given much help. The handicap was called "infant psychosis" and was thought to be caused by traumatic experiences. In her youth, my mother-in-law worked in childcare. She told me that autistic children were called mutes then. No one believed that they could learn to speak.

Lucas continues to blow his nose straight into the air, and he pees his pants several times a day. I can't wash all his clothes in time and have to buy more to keep pace. I'm worried about him. I speak with Carl, and we decide to locate other parents who've used Örjan's training method in order to find out more about their experiences. I call the parents of the boy who was completely cured after training with behavioral therapy and wonder if we might visit them. They invite us over for dinner. They live across the street from our office in the city. Sometimes, it's a small world.

We have pizza together. They tell us about their son and how he had begun speaking when he was little. Then his speech disappeared and he retreated into his own world. They began with behavioral therapy and were very careful to practice at least thirty hours a week. His preschool was positive, and everyone took an active part. They trained intensively for several years, both at preschool and at home, and the boy made enormous progress. They speak about that time as an illness and the present as him being cured. When he started school, he was like any other boy, and he had no autism spectrum symptoms left. We meet their son, who's at home playing with a friend. There is no noticeable difference between them, and he speaks the same as other children.

His mother says that she's constantly worried that the illness will return. She has her eye on him all the time and doesn't let him retreat into his own world. She wants to verify that he's keeping up with his lessons and isn't daydreaming, so she interrogates him every day about what he's done, and he must be able to explain. She usually double-checks with his teacher that it's correct. It feels like the boy is being monitored and isn't free, and that gives me the creepy feeling that his parents have taken over his life. When Carl and I are left alone for a while, I whisper to him how I feel, but he thinks I'm overreacting and projecting things that aren't there.

They're very helpful and lend us material that their son used in his training, even several binders of exercises they've done. We also borrow a video, a taped TV program from the United States called *The Nature of Things*. The program is about autism and ABA—applied behavior analysis, which is what the Lovaas method is called in the US. The film begins by describing how autistic children are different from other children. It shows how normal kids, kids with Down's syndrome, and autistic kids react in different situations. The situations are contrived and the participants are a child, its mother, and a psychologist. In the first scene, a girl of about one and a half years of age is sitting next to her mother at a table. A female psychologist is sitting across from them. She holds a ball in her hand, playing with it. Then she rolls the ball to the child, who catches it, makes eye contact with the psychologist, and rolls it back to her. In spite of the child's early age, interplay has started. The boy with Down's syndrome reacts the same way, but the autistic boy doesn't acknowledge the psychologist and plays with the ball by himself, not opening up for interplay. The film explains that this is an example of "joint attention." Very early, children show signs of having this ability, wanting to share their experiences with others. This is something autistic children lack. They experience things on their own and don't seem to understand or need to share their experiences with others.

In another scene, the psychologist sits and plays at hammering pegs. Suddenly, you see her hit her thumb. She yelps, and it looks as if she's in real pain. Both the normal child and the child with Down's syndrome look worried and show empathy for the psychologist. The autistic boy doesn't seem to notice that the psychologist has hurt herself, and instead takes the hammer and begins to examine it and strike the table with it. This is an example of "theory of mind." Autistic children are said to have difficulty understanding that others have thoughts, feelings, and needs.

In the last scene, the child, mother, and psychologist are sitting in their chairs, which have been placed in a semicircle. A little robot comes rolling across the floor toward them. The psychologist and mother show clear signs of being afraid of the object. The normal child watches how the adults behave, sees that they're frightened, and starts to cry. The boy with Down's syndrome watches the adults and then runs quickly up to the robot and kicks it until it falls over. The autistic boy doesn't watch the adults but goes up to the robot, picks it up, and begins to examine it. This situation shows how most children have basic survival instincts. They interpret situations by reading and mirroring how others react, something autistic children don't do. Autistic children don't learn that way, since they don't notice other people's reactions.

In this way the film demonstrates how autistic children live in their own world, and it goes on to show how you need to disturb them and break their isolation in order for them to notice other people and the world they share. It portrays the cases of several different kids who have worked with ABA. The children were first documented before they began the treatment. They didn't speak, flapped their hands, walked on their toes, and resorted to meaningless play, like just tossing things around the room. Then the film shows how the exercises work and how the children had developed after two or three years. They had all made enormous progress. One boy was declared cured and began attending a normal school. I recognize the training that's being depicted, except the trainers are curt in their tone and sometimes brusque, which makes me think of dog training. When the child succeeds, the trainers are unnaturally positive, in an exaggerated way that strikes me as fake.

I think the film is good anyway, until I get to a scene that makes me sit up in my chair. A five-year-old boy is going to practice having a normal conversation with his father. The boy has had an earbud fastened on his ear. The scene is played out in the kitchen. The father has just returned from the store and comes in carrying a large brown paper bag in his arms. He sets it down on the kitchen counter, and the boy enters the kitchen. Behind a corner, you can see a woman with a walkie-talkie. The father says something to the boy, and the woman hears what he says and whispers a sentence into the walkie-talkie, which the boy hears and then repeats verbatim to his father. The conversation continues for a while in the same fashion until they're finished, then the woman enters, rewards the boy, and tells him he's done a good job.

"Well said!" she says.

It's this scene that scares me. Is that the way I want Lucas to be? A little remote-controlled robot who learns things on command, without any possibility of thinking for himself and developing his own personality? It makes me afraid that we'll steer him too much with this training, that we'll brainwash him.

I also meet another mother whose child has worked with ABA. Her boy hasn't succeeded as well, but she's convinced he wouldn't have learned to speak at all if it hadn't been for this training program. She's from the United States, and she's taught her son English. He doesn't know any Swedish, but he understands and speaks English, in a slightly robot-like manner, she says. He doesn't say much, but he answers when spoken to.

Our kids usually get candy on Saturdays. Lucas loves chocolate, especially M&M's. Sara isn't fond of candy. She often eats only a little and leaves the rest. Lucas eats it all at once and usually confiscates Sara's leftovers as well.

One evening, after dinner, they each receive a small plastic bowl of M&M's. The kids watch a movie and then I take them off to bed. When they've gone to sleep, I go down to the kitchen. On the way, I pass the living room and see their candy bowls on the coffee table. In both the bowls, there are a few candies left, and all of them are red. I find that strange.

"Carl, come here," I call.

"What is it?"

"Come down here. I want to show you something."

He comes down from upstairs.

"Look!" I say and point to the bowls.

"What?"

"Don't you see? There are only red M&M's left."

"Yeah, maybe they didn't like them."

I taste a candy and it tastes the same as usual. Nothing wrong at all.

"No, it tastes fine."

"Well, maybe they just didn't want any more."

"Lucas always eats up his share. Why would he leave it now and why only the red ones?"

"Isn't it a good thing that he doesn't eat it all at once?" says Carl.

"Of course, but why do you think he only left the red ones?"

"I dunno," he answers.

"I think it has something to do with the color," I say. "We're working on colors now. We've begun with red, and it's been very slow going. Fredrik has brought M&M's into the exercises. I think maybe Lucas is not eating them because they remind him of the exercises."

"Do you really think so?" Carl asks.

"Yes, isn't that terrible! M&M's have always been something Lucas loves, and now there's negative conditioning and he avoids them."

"How is that possible?" Carl asks me. "What are they doing when they train him?"

I explain how Fredrik has held up different candies and asked about red, and when Lucas has answered correctly, he's received a candy, otherwise not. Since he's had problems with the exercise and hasn't learned the color, it's surely been very frustrating for him when Fredrik has sat there, waving his favorite candy in front of his nose. Sometimes he's allowed to taste it and sometimes not. He probably hasn't understood what he's supposed to do to get it.

"We don't know if that's true," says Carl. "I think we should try giving him some M&M's tomorrow and see what he does."

After dinner the next day, we give Lucas a bowl of M&M's. We study him on the sly and watch in horror as he eats all the candies except the red ones. If Lucas won't eat the candy he loves best, we've committed a terrible crime.

I thought it would just be his motivation for the training, but instead it turned into a negative force. Now it felt as if I had taken on the role of "God" in my child's life. I'm managing his inner motivation and am affecting and altering his behavior.

Just as Pavlov's dogs were made to drool when they heard a bell, I had made Lucas abhor red M&M's and changed his love for them into avoidance. This is awful. I'm frightened, afraid I'll hurt my own child, that I'll control him too much, that I'll eradicate his self-respect and identity. If his autistic behavior is contributing to his isolation, and it's difficult to understand his surroundings, what will happen if we mess with the few things he feels safe with, the things he thinks and feels on his own? How much more chaotic would the world be when he can't even trust his own feelings?

Added to the symptoms of stress Lucas has been manifesting, the red M&M's are the straw that breaks the camel's back. Behavioral training has been transformed into a negative force, dangerous to my child, since it messes with his psyche. We must make a decision. We cannot continue with this training. I can't defend it anymore; I don't want to experiment with my child's thoughts and wishes.

I inform Fredrik, Lotta, and my mother-in-law that we have to discontinue the program in its present form. I tell them about the candies and that I believe we're too controlling. I want to give Lucas more space to grow and have the opportunity to express his own personality. We need to rethink this. To find another strategy for his training. They ask me how that will happen, and I answer that I don't know, but that I'll work on it.

This worries my mother-in-law. She feels I'm making a sudden change of direction and not thinking of Lucas's best interests. Slowly, she has begun to accept that Lucas is late in his development, possibly autistic, and that he needs help to develop. When I first told her about the behavioral therapy, she was very skeptical, because it's intensive and demands a lot of the child, and she felt its attitude toward the child was hard. Now that we've begun training, she's changed her mind and thinks it gives Lucas a greater structure. She can also see that he's making progress.

For me, it's not a sudden change. For a while now, I've had a feeling that we've chosen the wrong method, and I've been grappling with the thought that we may be doing something that's damaging to our child, but to my mother-in-law it seems as if I was making things up. I try to explain that all I want is what's best for Lucas. If I don't believe in something, then we can't continue. Nothing stays still, you need to constantly watch, question, and evaluate what you're doing. Especially when it's your own child. I'm afraid that it's dangerous to continue along this path, but she can't understand why.

I get into a heated discussion with Lotta. She doesn't know how to react. She knows this method, and this is how she wants to work with Lucas. I say that I don't know how we can continue, but that I have a few thoughts about the method. Unfortunately, we can't find a solution together, and in the end, she leaves us. It's no fun to lose Lotta, because she's a good teacher, but if she can't innovate, there's no room for her anymore. I need to look out for my child's best interests, for Lucas.

I exist in a vacuum. I put all my energy into finding a method that can help my child to develop. I thought behavioral therapy was a good method. Lucas was making progress, and I had let go, left the responsibility to someone else. What will we do now, when I no longer believe in this method? When I realized that Lucas was autistic and understood his difficulties, the ground disappeared from beneath my feet, and I fell into a deep hole. From there, we had crawled up until we were on top of the mountain and saw the sky and a future for our son, but now I've lost my foothold once again and fallen into the abyss. I'm groping in the dark. There's no light anywhere. How will we find a new path?

MY OWN METHOD

I have to start over from the beginning. Again, I must take on the role of my child's teacher. I must find a new way for us to train Lucas. He needs training to develop, but how should it be structured? I decide to create an educational plan. To do that, I first need to assess what Lucas knows and can do successfully, so I can then see which difficulties he has and what he needs to work on.

ABA has been a very good start for Lucas, since it has given him the ability to respond when we speak to him. Behavioral therapy has helped us teach him to sit down at a table, concentrate, listen, understand, and do various exercises, and he really surprised us. When we showed him pictures and he learned to point out things that we asked him about, we noticed what a huge passive vocabulary he has. He knew almost every noun and verb that we presented to him. When he saw the pictures, he began to say the words. The pictures give him some stimulus and are a good support while he develops his speech.

He had more knowledge than we thought, but since he doesn't speak himself or make himself understood, we had no idea. The first speech therapist we went to lacked the tools to test him. She couldn't get him to answer any of the questions she asked and couldn't do an assessment of him either.

The core of Lucas's problem is communication. He doesn't seem to understand what it's for. When he does use words, they often lack a communicative purpose, and when he says a word to communicate, he often chooses the wrong one, meaning something different than what he wants to say. The need to communicate with others is hard to motivate for someone who doesn't see the advantages of it. I want to show Lucas the functions of language and what joy it can give him to use it. I want to show him that, using language, he can receive things, have wishes fulfilled, and get appreciation and sympathy, and that he can develop his own ideas and take them a step further.

If he doesn't learn to communicate, he'll cease to develop. To learn new things, he must have some benefit from other people or books and films, and then he must be able to understand what's said and meant. Otherwise, Lucas will live in his own little bubble. What a dull life he'll have if he doesn't learn to communicate so he can participate in our world.

I develop exercises with which he'll experience the feeling of being able to steer and affect someone else. We play in the big bed. I tickle, chase, and wrestle with him, which he loves. I teach him words and phrases, for example, "Fall down." When he says, "Fall down," I fall all over the bed and he screams with laughter. I want him to feel that it's fun and show him that, with language, he can get me to do things that he thinks are funny. I want him to feel empowered by language and the joy of being able to speak and be involved with others.

I surf the Web, and in the US I find image banks for sale, developed to help autistic children with language. With the images, I can teach Lucas language concepts like nouns, prepositions, comparatives, adjectives, adverbs, and much more. By using the pictures and then generalizing into our everyday life, I want him to increase his comprehension. I also find picture programs at the autism center.

I read about communication alternatives to speech and find a tool called VocaFlex, a voice output communication aid, which is a device used by individuals who are either unable to speak or whose speech is unintelligible, and I manage to order it through the autism center. It's a blue plastic box that works like a kind of tape player, with multiple buttons on which you can put various image overlays. A picture overlay consists of sixteen small images. I can choose which pictures I want to use and record a text for each picture. Then, by pressing the picture with a finger, the message is activated. I make an overlay containing pictures that express the following:

I'm hungry.
I'm thirsty.
I want to have ice cream.
I want to have a sandwich.
I want to have a Coke.
I want to watch TV.
I want to ride in the car.
I'm angry.
I want to see Grandma.
I want to swim in the pool.
I want to play.
I want to jump on the bed.
I want to get a hug.
I want to read a book.
I want to sleep.
I want to dance.

So now Lucas can press a button and hear the sentence that goes with the picture. I make another overlay with songs and yet another with colors. I've thought about doing something else too; when Lucas starts preschool, I can take pictures of the kids and personnel and then record their names with the pictures. In that way, he can learn everyone's name.

The VocaFlex is mainly intended as a tool to stimulate language, not to replace it. I want Lucas to be able to use it when he wants to say various things but also to be able to press buttons and listen to different songs. I want to awaken his interest in speech and singing, and I want him to think it's exciting.

I also consider harnessing the computer as an aid in communication. We're already working with various simple computer programs that

Lucas likes. I find a program called Widgit SymWriter, which is for writing with symbols, and, while writing, you hear the item read aloud through a speech synthesizer or recorded speech. By pressing different symbols or typing text on the keyboard, you can make sentences that you can hear and see on the screen in the form of images and texts. There are already pictures in the program, but you can also use your own photos of people and places and other things to communicate about. Since Lucas is visually oriented, I figure that this could be a way to make the structure of language available to him. For the time being, I feel it's too advanced for him, but it's something that I want to start doing when he's come a little further along in his communication.

I take a course focusing on the importance of play for social interplay. The teachers show how you can get autistic kids to participate by using simple party games. Games are good, because they have rules that give them structure, which makes it easier for autistic children while also nurturing their social interaction.

I try playing a very simple game with Lucas. We sit on small chairs, facing each other at his table. Some colorful wooden blocks and a plastic plate are on the table. I put on a cap to mark that it's my turn, take a block, and put it on the plastic plate. I place the cap on Lucas's head to clearly show that it's his turn and say, "Now it's your turn," then help him pick out a block and put it on top of mine. Then I take the cap and put it on my head and stack another block on top of the tower.

We take turns building a tall tower. It sways some from time to time and finally crashes down. Lucas claps his hands with glee. I show Sara how to do this, and then there are three of us playing the building block game. It's a very simple game, but a great way to learn taking turns while doing something fun together. Through play and games, I would like to develop Lucas's interplay and communication skills, not through correction when he's made mistakes, as in the training program.

I also read more about various kinds of play therapy, in spite of the fact that I had rejected it earlier. We have small finger puppets at home. There's a royal family, with a king, queen, prince, and princess, precisely the same number of people as in our family. With Sara, I try to enact different situations with the puppets. I give them our names, and she quickly grasps who is who. I create different situations, and she plays along. She speaks fluently, though she isn't two yet. It's interesting to listen to what she says and try to interpret what she means, but I understand that it's hopeless to try something similar with Lucas. He hasn't reached that level yet.

MY THOUGHTS BEGIN TO SPIN FASTER AND FASTER

At night, I sit in our office up in the attic and read theories of child language development. Babies gurgle, prattle, imitate sounds, say single words, which they later begin to combine. They turn to other people and communicate, but they also talk to themselves. I study my daughter, who is a little over one and a half. Her monologues are games that reflect reality and affirm her identity. She sits in the bathtub, talking to her doll about washing and diving and splashing in the water. She also talks a lot about herself and what she's going to do.

Monologue is an important step in developing a dialogue. You need to be able to put your own thoughts into words before you can communicate them. Very young kids talk to themselves, expressing their thoughts aloud, and eventually learn to think silently. People who are designated as high-function autistics, which many equate with Asperger syndrome, often mumble to themselves until a late age. Theories suggest that this is a late, drawn-out monologue that they've never learned to quiet or keep to themselves. The step after audible monologues is formulating your thoughts silently. Lucas hardly says a word and never monologues. How will he be able to have a dialogue with another person if he never talks to himself?

Everyone around a tiny baby is attuned to interpreting the baby's signals and efforts to communicate, and to responding. A baby may believe that its surroundings are all-encompassing, understanding and knowing everything, but when the child grows, it begins to become a person in its own right, develops its ego, and separates from others. It's possible that Lucas hasn't even come as far as understanding that he's a separate person.

When I study Lucas, I get the idea that he believes that I, his mother, and possibly everyone else too, experiences what he does, that we know and feel precisely what he knows and feels. Maybe he believes that what he experiences in his head is what everyone else experiences, a dizzying thought. Because, if that's accurate, he can't understand the need to communicate; there's no need to talk if everyone around him already has the same information that he has. It that's true, why even try to communicate? Totally unnecessary. What if that's what's going on? How am I to know? It's impossible to find out. I decide to be extra clear in different situations and try to explain to Lucas that I don't know what he wants to have or to do, that he must tell me in words, so I'll understand.

Lucas doesn't use many words, and I'm afraid we read too much into his attempts to communicate. His grandmother means well, but I think she puts words in his mouth—her words, not his. I often feel she's misinterpreting him, imposing her own ideas rather than intuiting what Lucas wants or knows. I want to give him more space, greater opportunity to be heard and I want us to hear accurately what he has to say.

It's important to separate your own feelings from those of the other person, to prevent your comprehension from becoming just a projection of your personal feelings and needs. I don't want us to superimpose *our* words on Lucas's thoughts and feelings, because in that case we may just be projecting our own assumptions and wishes in various situations. Instead, we should try in every way imaginable to get Lucas to tell or show his thoughts to us. We must provide the right conditions for his success, or he'll lose any faith in communicating before he's learned to do it. Since he doesn't speak, this is difficult, but he uses some body language, which we try to understand, and in order to do that we ask Lucas questions that he can be expected to understand. At the very least, he can answer yes or no.

As I see it, the responsibility for communication rests with the person who has a command of it. It's this person's job to find out what the true meaning is in any exchange. That's the person with the tools to communicate. The person with the handicap is doing his or her best as it is. The person with the greater ability can always ask questions to find out what the other person means.

When I have a conversation about this with my mother-in-law, she tells me how her father was struck with aphasia at a young age, after an aneurism. She tells me about bringing her fiancé home for the first time and introducing him to her father, who was lying in the hospital bed. Her father tried to say something, but no one understood him; in the end, he was weeping in frustration. If you can't express yourself, you will be a prisoner in your own body.

I'm afraid that if Lucas doesn't develop language, either spoken or by some alternative means of communication, the gap between what Lucas wants to communicate and what he succeeds in saying will lead to enormous frustration, which can, in turn, lead to behavioral problems.

The urge to express oneself and be understood is powerful. I attended a lecture where a father told of his autistic teenage daughter. A couple of years previously, he and his family rented a summer cabin, and last summer they did again. On the way there, in the car, the daughter had a temper tantrum and began kicking and flailing in the back seat. They tried to calm her, but it went as far as her kicking out the car window. They pulled over to the side of the road and stopped. The girl immediately jumped out of the car, stood in the road, and pointed at the gas station they had passed. Bells began to ring for the parents, who recalled that they had stopped at that very gas station to buy ice cream the previous summer. She remembered, and she wanted an ice cream, but she hadn't been able to make her parents understand. They got into the car, turned around, and went back. The girl ran into the station and chose the ice cream she wanted.

The father told us that now they use photographs to communicate, and suddenly his daughter has access to a language that she previously lacked. Her outbursts and behavior problems have decreased dramatically. The frustration of not being able to get her message out had increased with age. It's clear, we must help Lucas now. I realize that it's important to train early, and I know the reasons why.

All the speech therapists and the others we saw during the evaluation have been surprised that Lucas seems to be such a happy boy. I think it's because he doesn't feel frustrated, since he can now make himself somewhat understood. If you don't get feedback for your wishes, you lose the desire to communicate, and that is what I believe happened about a year ago when Lucas was two. Maybe we just didn't understand what he wanted. His attempts to reach us were fruitless, and he retired, gave up, and isolated himself. He withdrew to live in his own world.

I want to create an educational plan for Lucas, so I need to identify his strengths and weaknesses. When I observe his behavior, I reflect on myself and how I function in the world. It occurs to me that I may have certain autistic characteristics. My speech wasn't delayed, but sometimes I have difficulty finding words and discussing things directly. It takes a long time for me to put my thoughts into words. It's easier for me to write down my thoughts than to voice them.

My mother described a few episodes from my childhood. Once, I was at the zoo with my grandmother. We had walked around the whole day and looked at the animals. When I came home and took off my shoes, my feet were bloody. My grandmother was shocked that I hadn't said anything, limped, or let her know in some way that I had blisters. When my mother told me this, she said that I was always such a brave little girl.

Body language is the second form of communication that humans use to express their desires and emotions. Autistic people often have badly developed body language, and maybe the reason for that is they aren't good at communicating in the first place, so they don't intuit and develop a body language. People within the autism spectrum often have difficulty with or no skill at all in deciphering what a person is saying through facial expressions or other bodily gestures. Another difficulty they have is asking for help, since, for that, you have to turn to another person, but they don't understand the point of interplay and communication. Autistic children are said to have a high pain threshold. However, is that really true, or is it because they don't know how to tell us when they are in pain? Have they really examined the children's pain threshold? I notice that Lucas hardly ever cries or tells me if he has hurt himself.

I've never considered myself handicapped, but I have felt alienated. I grew up with my mother and my two sisters. They always called me normal because I never showed strong emotions. They probably thought I was a little cold, since I don't express strong feelings or empathize with others. I don't get envious, and I don't feel schadenfreude. I seldom get angry, and if someone treats me unfairly I cry, but more because I can't give a quick retort than because I am angry.

I believe that women with autistic spectrum disorders are able to compensate to a higher degree than men are. Women and men communicate differently. Research shows that women use both sides of the brain more than men do when communicating. That may be why more men than women receive a diagnosis of autism, but it's also possible that autism in women isn't as pronounced as it is in men and for that reason they aren't diagnosed as often.

Maybe there is something valid in the theory of cold mothers who cause their children's autism. Not that autism is a direct result of the way a child is treated, but rather that there may be a genetic factor. I mean that the mothers could have similar problems themselves. Maybe I'm a cold mother, but not because I lack feelings for my children, but because my own ability to communicate is faulty, which, in turn, might affect my capacity for emotional communication. Carl and I both feel that we display some autistic symptoms, and we've wondered whether Lucas could have inherited his autism from us. Carl is verbal, which doesn't synchronize with autism, but he has total focus, leading him to put all else aside. We are both mathematically inclined and studied natural sciences. Carl went on to become an engineer, and I became an economist.

Some researchers believe that autistic people have memory disorders. We humans use our memory almost constantly. We rely on memory for everything from learning new things to remembering the way home. In a lecture I attended, Gunilla Gerland, a highly functional autistic woman in Sweden who is also a world-famous author, described how she developed strategies to get by in her daily life. When she was in school, she couldn't find her way to the cafeteria, and she had problems recognizing her classmates' faces. When it was time for lunch, she noted what the girl in the seat in front of her was wearing. Then she kept a lookout for those clothes and followed them to the cafeteria.

Episodic memory, where we store experiences, is the most aberrant in autistic people. Disturbances in episodic memory make it difficult to remember things that you have personally experienced. Sharing memories, for example intimate details about your past, is an important skill to have when connecting socially with others. Semantic memory, on the other hand, which is of facts, meanings, and concepts, seems to function fine for people on the spectrum and they remember information they've read or seen more easily than autobiographical memories.

I think about my own memory. I've always had a hard time remembering my own experiences and have been impressed when other people recount detailed descriptions of theirs. I have difficulty producing images from memory. It feels like my hard drive has been erased. It's just blank. I used to wonder whether my experiences just weren't vivid enough for my brain to be able to store them.

I've always made sure to take photos of things that I've done and to put them in albums. Maybe that's been a way to compensate for my bad memory. Without memories, you have no past. My life is in photo albums. I am there in the photos, and when I look at them, I know what I've done, but I still don't remember any details. It's also hard for me to find my way back to places I've already been, but I usually have a map in my handbag or in the car.

I study and analyze Lucas, comparing how he communicates to the way his little sister and we, his parents, do, and my thoughts become increasingly theoretical. Normal children engage in two-way communication as soon as a couple of hours after birth, but Lucas never has. I see in Lucas a kind of communication but only one-way. He sends messages but doesn't respond. I begin to think about him maybe having communicated in a way that I haven't been able to read. He doesn't understand the meaning of a social interaction. Is he living in a physical world instead of a social one, a world where things and objects have a greater significance than people? Maybe he communicates through physical actions instead of using eye contact, miming, gestures, and sounds, like ordinary people? Maybe kicking off his blanket instead of screaming was his way of telling us he was hungry?

I'm afraid that I've misinterpreted his attempts to communicate. What if he has had a different way of communicating since birth, a physical approach that I failed to recognize? For many years then, I've been hindering his growth rather than supporting it, which has resulted in Lucas switching off his communication instead of developing it.

I saw Lucas, the autistic child, as a transmitter from the moment he was born. Normal children are both sending and receiving messages. Lucas lacked the capacity for two-way interaction. He sent messages to me; I tried to answer in the way I believed he would understand, but I received nothing in response.

Before you can interact with your surroundings, you must also be able to receive messages. That's something I think autistic kids have trouble doing on their own, and that's where they need help. When they succeed in making that connection, their development takes off, but only then. I feel that I've found the core problem in autism—the inability to grasp two-way communication.

I liken Lucas to a blinking lighthouse. It only sends out messages but cannot respond. On the contrary, it signals, "Keep away." I look at the criteria for autism and see that they all can be derived in different ways from the lack of two-way communication. The criteria are only symptoms that appear because the autistic person doesn't have the basics for communication. A diagnosis of autism is based on the following three areas:

1. Qualitative impairment in social interaction
    The main part of this disturbance seems to be the lack of social contacts with other people. People with autism show a lack of interest in sharing joys and interests with others, or in participating with others in games and common pursuits.

Lucas wants to play and share experiences. He loves to wrestle in bed or play tag and likes to swim in our pool with us. In those contexts, he understands and can participate on his own terms, with one-way interaction. I believe that autistic people *are* interested in social interaction, but they don't know the rules, don't understand how, and don't know what to do to approach others in interplay. On top of that, if your language abilities remain undeveloped, it's very hard to have social contact with other people.

2. Qualitative impairment in communication
    People with autism have disturbances in communication. Previously, half of all autistic people failed to develop spoken language. Now, these numbers are smaller, due to access to better training. Many of those who speak use echoing (repeating what the other person says). It is difficult for a person with autism to interpret facial expressions and gestures and to use these to communicate.

If a person doesn't understand two-way communication, it's very hard to develop functional language, one built on sending and receiving messages, and you won't understand body language, which is also a form of communication.

3. Limited powers of imagination
The autistic person is strongly preoccupied with one or more stereotyped, narrow, or odd interests, in a manner that is abnormal in intensity or content. Many adhere inflexibly to certain routines and rituals. Some are very preoccupied with parts of objects or use them in abnormal ways.

I don't believe that autistic people have limited imaginations, but they can have difficulty expressing their imagination, since they don't communicate very well. Temple Grandin, a highly functional autistic woman, says that she was the one who came up with the craziest pranks in school.

We all want control over our lives and circumstances, and we all have rituals and routines. Most adults use a calendar. Many of us follow set morning routines. Some of us must have a cup of coffee before we can start the day. We may have different bad habits, which could be called rituals, such as biting the top of a pen or twisting a lock of hair when we're contemplating what to write. Autistic people also acquire rituals and routines, though these differ from those of other people because autistics haven't reached as far in their development.

In the ABA method of training, communication was limited. I asked Lucas to perform an action and he did it, but then the dialogue was interrupted in order to move on to a new exercise. Research shows that one of the most difficult things for autistic people to do is to initiate communication. My theory is that I must teach Lucas to have a conversation, to both initiate and respond, in order to succeed in maintaining one.

I want to teach Lucas two-way communication, to be a trans-mitter-receiver-transmitter. I want to do it by keeping the dialogue alive, asking follow-up questions when he answers, to trigger him to respond to me, so that he'll need to take me into consideration. I build the dialogue around his physical needs, like hunger, thirst, and sleep, and his emotional needs, such as the fun he experiences when we do things together. I want him to feel like "the boss" and to show him that it's fun to be able to affect your environment in various ways.

My hypothesis is that if you can just teach children two-way interaction and develop their understanding of the need to respond and react from their own conceptual world, they will be able to develop normally instead of withdrawing and developing autism. If they go through life in one-way interactions, they will develop autism, with behavioral and emotional disturbances as effects. Hasn't anyone thought about this before? I feel that I've hit on a scoop, the solution to the autism problem. . . .

My thoughts are crystal clear, and I see clearly which way we should go.

Sender – Receiver – Sender
S – R – S
S – R – S
S – R – S

During the day, I perform everyday tasks, go to the open daycare with Sara, and take turns with Fredrik training Lucas. At night, I sit in the attic and read books. I'm barely sleeping at all, perhaps a couple of hours a night. I scribble my thoughts, which become long essays. My discourse is increasingly intellectual, and I send my analyses via email to my mother-in-law. She answers as best she can, but I don't think she understands what I mean.

From studying autism and communication, I change to more philosophical and psychological questions. With Fredrik, I discuss Plato and Socrates.

I analyze how we think and act, and conclude that all people have dual personalities—one side is rational and the other emotional.

We each have a different combination of these two factors, which is the basis of our personalities.

If you draw a curve for normal distribution, rational thinking on one side and emotional thinking on the other, most people are somewhere in the middle. I see that all people within the autism spectrum, including myself and even my husband, are at the rational thinking end of the curve.

If this is accurate, then autism is not an illness but rather a personality characteristic. My mother-in-law is at the opposite end of the curve from me, which I believe is one of the reasons it's so hard for us to understand each other.

When I don't get the feedback I expect from her, I involve my father-in-law in my theoretical discussion, hoping he can explain to my mother-in-law what I mean. He is more rational than emotional.

It's important to me to communicate my stance, since it's about our son and how we need to treat him. Naturally, I discuss all this with Carl, and I succeed in getting him to understand what I mean. I'm so convincing in my reasoning that he thinks I've gotten closer to the cure for autism, something researchers have sought for years. My thoughts ricochet inside my head like a pinball being kept in the game and never rolling down.

But my mother-in-law doesn't understand me, and when I can't reach my father-in-law either, I call a family council. In the evening, when the kids are asleep, I gather Carl and my in-laws at our place. We sit in the living room and talk. They don't want to listen, to accept. They don't understand what I mean, and I feel dismayed that I can't reach them. When the words aren't enough, I fetch my written notes to have some support. They think I'm progressing too swiftly, that I lack strong support for my decisions, while I think they're too careful, conservative, and afraid of change. I make parallels to when I initially wanted to get them to accept that Lucas was different. They couldn't see then, either, what was obvious to me. Instead, they had accused me of making things up.

I'm standing in the middle of the circle, and the stones are coming from all directions.

They hit me with full force.

I try to ward them off, but it hurts too much.

I run off, crying, when they still don't want to understand.

THE BOUNDARY
BETWEEN DREAM AND
REALITY DISAPPEARS

I feel no hunger or fatigue. In the evenings, when the kids have gone to sleep, I sit up until 3:00 a.m. reading. Then I go to bed and wake up at five, ready to go. I often dream something about what I read the previous evening and awaken with new angles. I immediately get out of bed, sit down, and write my thoughts. My brain is never at rest. Thoughts have the speed of light. Wherever I am, I need to write down what I'm thinking because the thoughts are fleeting and I'm afraid they'll disappear. Even while I'm driving, I keep a notepad next to me so I can jot down ideas. When I stop at a red light, I can write long sentences, and I have the notepad on the steering wheel to write down the main points. Days pass, and my thoughts are drowning my brain, and soon it can no longer take in outer stimuli.

One day, I'm on my way home from town. I'm driving alone in my car, and I approach the Danvikstull drawbridge. Suddenly, I hear bells ringing. I look around and see that the drawbridge is opening and I just barely brake and stop in time before a road barrier cuts my car in two. I've driven past the first red light and nearly passed the second. My car is alone, in the front, closest to the bridge. The other drivers have stopped at the first red light. I see the bridge open before my eyes, and I understand that I can no longer drive.

I sleep even less. The boundary between dream and reality begins to disappear. One night I dream that my deceased father speaks to me and I wake believing he's still alive. A couple of months ago, it was ten years since he died in the car crash. I lie in bed, and my thoughts are spinning. Maybe he DIDN'T die in the crash? Maybe it was all fake? Maybe he wanted to start a new life somewhere and change his identity? If he had committed a crime, the statute of limitations would have expired by now, this year. How can I find him if he's alive? Where is he? How can I reach him? I figure, if he is alive, he must have access to the Internet. Maybe I can find him that way, try and find his email address and contact him. I get out of bed and go up to our office in the attic and sit down in front of my computer. I write down a list of possible email addresses he might have and start sending emails into cyberspace, but to my disappointment they all bounce back with the reply "User unknown." He died near a place called Jenny. Was that a sign? Are there other places with that name? I search Google Maps. In Surinam, a country in between Guyana and French Guyana in northeastern South America, I find a spot on the coast called Jenny. He loved South America. Of course, that's where he is.

A window has opened that was previously closed. My senses are sharpened, and I take in everything in my surroundings. People turn to me in a different manner than before. At the open preschool, where stay-at-home moms can bring very young children to meet and play together, everyone gathers around me. I'm the focal point, and I lead the discussion. Perhaps it has something to do with my viewpoint? I see everything and everyone and cannot leave well enough alone. Energy emanates from me in an almost supernatural way. Is it something that affects others unconsciously, or is it just my own experience? The feeling is so strong, and the energy surrounds all living things.

One day, I visit my friend Camilla, who lives in the neighborhood. We're going for coffee, and Sara has a play date with her daughter. I take the car and park in the driveway, lift Sara from her car seat, and put her on the ground. I take her small hand in mine, and we walk up to the house. Suddenly, Rex, their giant black German shepherd, comes bounding up. He's a little wild and usually runs around like crazy in the yard, but he's a good dog, and all he wants to do is play. I bend down, meet him, and look into his large, dark brown eyes. Immediately, he sits and becomes completely calm. Our gazes meet for a moment that seems like an eternity. We have a connection that flows between us like an invisible force. When I straighten up, he follows us closely and rubs against my legs. We ascend the stairs to the front door. I ring the bell and Rex sits, close by me.

Camilla opens the door.

"Hi, nice to see you," she says. "Come on in. Wow, Rex is so calm! What have you done to him?" she says with a laugh.

"Nothing," I answer, and smile secretively. "We just said our hellos."

Strange things begin to occur, and it scares me. A ceiling light in the hall by the living room begins to act strangely. When I'm in the vicinity, its luminosity increases and decreases, without my using the dimmer. At night, different toys begin to play, without my pressing any buttons to activate them. The telephone rings, but no one is there when I answer.

"Hello. Hello?"

All I hear are clicking sounds. No dial tone or voice.

When the children watch Cartoon Network or any other TV channel during the daytime, we have bad reception and can't watch. Suddenly, the transmission is interrupted and all we see is a snowstorm. It feels as if the air is charged with static electricity, and it's as if some supernatural force has taken over and is steering our lives, or at least trying to. If I put on a DVD, everything is normal again.

One night, when Sara wakes up, I lay down beside her and she falls back to sleep. I remain with her, thinking of different rules and stances we should adopt in our family. I feel that candy on Saturdays only is a stupid rule, mainly adopted to make it easy for parents instead of being for the benefit of the kids. If kids are allowed to have candy only on Saturdays, a practice that's very common in Sweden, it's easier for parents to handle their nagging and to refer to the fact that they'll get it on Saturday. I don't eat candy only on Saturdays, so why should they have to? I hug my little girl, sleeping peacefully beside me. She moves a little and talks in her sleep. I listen and hear her say, "Candy." Candy, I think. I was just lying there, thinking about Saturday candy. Can she read my thoughts in her unconscious? We are close, spend day and night together. Maybe small children, still developing a language, have a kind of sixth sense? Do they have telepathic abilities? Telepathy is a direct connection or contact between two sentient beings. It is the ability to read another person's thoughts or to transfer one's thoughts to another without the use of speech, signs, or other physical signals. I've read that there are researchers who believe that, millions of years ago, before we developed a language, people communicated with thoughts. Maybe telepathy is something that we all have when we're born, but the ability diminishes as we learn to speak?

Later, on the same day, I'm thinking: Lucas hasn't developed a spoken language. How are his telepathic abilities? What if he can read my thoughts? I worry about the terrible thoughts I've had and how they've affected him. I know that, when we began to suspect autism, Carl and I wondered if Lucas would ever be able to live a normal life with such a terrible handicap. It would be so limiting, so lonely. He would live in isolation, closed in his own world, and be very dependent upon others. It went so far that we thought, independently of each other, that it would've been better for Lucas if he died than needing to live such a horrible life. Death would be liberating, in comparison with life. We wished the life out of him, our little child. When I think this, I hear Lucas walking around sniffling the snot straight out into the air, one of his tics, like he usually does. He snorts, snorts and sniffles.

I can't see him, but I call out to him, "Lucas, stop snorting!"

However, he doesn't stop, and I go to find him. The little chubby three-year-old comes out of the bathroom, straight toward me. I see to my horror and despair that his nose is bleeding. Bright red blood is running from his nostrils down over his lips.

I start to cry, fall on my knees, and hug him.

"Forgive me Lucas, I'm sorry. We don't want any harm to come to you. We love you so much. We only want what's best for you. We want you to get well, to be able to talk with us. To be with us. Beloved child. You and Sara, you two mean the most to us. More than anything. You know that. You are everything to us."

After a while, I let go of him and get a Kleenex from my pocket. I carefully wipe his nose. My face is close to his and for once, our gazes meet. He looks at me with large, serious blue eyes, exactly as if he wants to say, "I know, Mom, I know."

I'm cold, in spite of all the warm sweaters I put on. At night, I can't sleep. When I close my eyes, I see pictures. Even in the day, when I close my eyes, I see symbols. It's as if my brain cannot relax. Impressions wash over me and leave me without peace. Everything must be interpreted, and I begin to read messages everywhere, in billboards, in ads from Pampers, in a TV show. A higher truth is touching my life and me.

One day, a black-and-white movie is on TV. It's *A Giant Swede: Harry Victor*. The main character is a kind of spy, and it suddenly occurs to me that my father was of course a spy. He worked for SÄPO, the Swedish Secret Police, or something like it. That's why he's gone underground and disappeared. What a brilliant, logical explanation! That's it.

Up in the attic, there are two rooms, the office, which is the white room, and our cinema, with black walls and floor. In the evening, I usually sit in the white room and Carl in the black. One evening, Carl is watching a movie, and I go in to say something to him about the dream I had of my father, that I believe he's still alive. The air feels heavy and electric.

When I sit on the couch and tell him, my eyeglasses fall off. One of the arms has come off because the screw that keeps my glasses together has fallen out. I pick them up and put them on again. They sit a little crooked, since one arm is missing. I continue to talk and almost immediately, one of my diamond earrings falls off. Without any rational explanation.

It feels ominous. What's happening? Is it my dad trying to communicate with me? Is he sending me a sign?

My husband is now beginning to worry that all is not right with me. The next day, he calls my sister, Eva, and asks her to come and sleep over. I try to tell her about our father and that I believe he's still alive, but she won't accept any of what I'm saying and tries to prove the opposite. We get nowhere, and in the evening she makes sure that we go to bed. I fall asleep, then wake up after a couple of hours, go upstairs, and sit in front of the computer again to search the world over for my missing father.

The next day, Carl wants to take me to lunch. He has arranged for his mother to come and babysit. We go to the Hotel Långholmen restaurant. Long ago, the hotel was a prison, built in the early nineteenth century. Before Carl and I moved in together, we spent a night in one of their rooms, as they call the cells. Maybe he wanted everything to be back to normal again, and that was why he brought me there, but I feel anything but normal.

It's late April, and the spring sun is shining from a blue sky. The outdoor section is closed, but I succeed in charming the waiter into letting us eat lunch outside. I'm not particularly hungry and order a salad and a glass of white wine. Carl has a shrimp sandwich. We lean against the building, and the sun is warming us nicely. I'm glad we're alone, because I'm restless and have difficulty sitting still. I go and fetch more bread and dressing. Later, I go to the restroom in order to keep moving.

After lunch, we get in the car and Carl drives. He doesn't drive homeward. He takes another road, over the Västerbro Bridge and on to Kungsholmen. We turn into a parking lot, close to a large building. In spite of my mental state, I still have one foot in reality, and I understand where we're headed. Carl parks. I open the car door, get out, and run away. Away from the parking lot, toward the green belt close by. I hide behind the trees. Carl runs after me. I feel hunted, like a wild animal being captured. Carl can't catch me and calls my sister Eva, who comes. Together, they wheedle and reason with me, and finally I follow them in, in to the psychiatric emergency ward at Saint Göran Hospital.

Upon entering, we pass a kiosk. I see the headlines, and it's as if every one of them has something important to tell me. I sneak away from Carl and Eva and approach the woman in the kiosk, asking for one copy of each of the newspapers they sell. She starts putting together a bundle, and they arrive and stop her just before I try to pay.

We see a doctor. Carl and Eva tell him about my background. He asks if I've had similar problems previously.

Eva says that I had hyperthyroidism many years ago. Hyperthyroidism is when the thyroid gland is overactive and produces excess thyroid hormones. This makes the body's functions speed up and leads to symptoms such as shaking, weight loss, and anxiety. It increases your metabolism and your body goes into overdrive. I had heart palpitations, heightened pulse, sweats, shakes, was irritated, restless, and easily upset. I also lost a lot of weight. Eva thinks my symptoms remind her of those. Once the doctor has observed and spoken with me, he concludes this is not an overactive thyroid. He believes I'm suffering from a psychosis. Carl and Eva want to take me home with some sleeping pills, but the doctor thinks otherwise. Against my own and my family's will, I am committed in accordance with Swedish law to compulsory psychiatric treatment. I receive Stesolid and Nitrazepam. I fall asleep and stay that way for fourteen hours.

WARD 22

The next day, I'm moved to the hospital a stone's throw from where we live. I'm admitted to Ward 22, which is on the top floor, maybe so it won't be easy to escape. The door is locked and can be opened only by the caregivers. The ward consists of a long corridor, with rooms on both sides. The women are separated from the men, but there are both in this ward. There are dormitories for multiple persons but also private rooms. A few rooms are group therapy rooms and treatment rooms. The cafeteria functions as a day room as well, and there's a couch and TV. That room has lots of daylight, and, from the tables by the windows, you have a view of the area for miles. I can almost see our home. At the end of the corridor, there's a smaller day room. You can listen to the radio there, and there's a TV that doesn't work. Halfway down the corridor, there's a smoking room, shared by patients and staff alike.

I'm placed in a dormitory with three other women. Next to each bed, there's a small screen, so the patients can have some privacy.

From the medical records:

At our meeting, the patient is very closed off. Quite correct behavior, formally. Describes the occurrences of the last few days and their son's illness initially in our conversation quite correctly and adequately, eventually beginning to slide into many associations about the possibility of treatment where she herself has found a way to teach the children to communicate. Quite emotionally unstable during most of our talk. Laughs inaptly and is close to tears alternately. Doesn't want to stay at the hospital, feels no need of care. Needs to go home and needs the support of her family.

My thoughts are spinning, and I try to put them down on paper. I talk to everyone and try to explain what I mean. At night, when everyone has gone to bed, I talk to myself. The first night, I sleep for three or four hours, in spite of the sleeping pills. I receive stronger medication and then start having trouble speaking. It feels uncomfortable. I feel strange, like I'm among strangers. I feel insecure. I want to go to my sister's place and rest up there, to be with someone who knows me and likes me. I don't want to stay in this place.

Carl comes to visit me every day. We have conversations with the doctor. I tell them that I want to leave here, that I don't want medicine. The doctor says that I must stay until I'm better. He thinks I need the medication, and reluctantly I agree to it, despite the fact that it makes me feel very uneasy.

It's the fifth morning in a row that I wake up early. It's 3:00 a.m., and I can't get back to sleep. I don't want to be here anymore. I want to go home. I want to talk to Carl. After an hour, I go out into the hallway and over to the telephone to call him. One of the night personnel hears me and sticks his head into the corridor.

"You can't call now. It's four o'clock in the morning," he says.

"I want to talk to my husband."

"You'll have to wait until eight o'clock."

"He won't mind if I wake him up."

"It's the middle of the night. You can't call now."

"I don't care." I want to call Carl and begin dialing the number.

He walks up to me, hangs up the phone, takes me by the arm, and leads me back to my room.

"Go back to sleep. You can call in the morning."

I go back into my room. I really need to hear Carl's voice, to speak with him. I have to tell him that I don't want to be here any longer and I want to come home. I stand by the door, listening.

I need to talk to Carl, to feel that someone cares about me, knows I'm here, and acknowledges my existence. Once it's quiet outside again, I sneak out to the telephone. I am just about to lift the receiver when I hear him opening the door and entering the hallway.

He walks toward me.

"I want to call!" I cry.

"You can't do it now."

He moves closer. I feel desperate; I really want to hear Carl's voice.

"Go away! Leave me alone!"

"You'll have to wait a few hours."

"No, I want to call now. I don't want to wait a few hours. He won't be home. Now I know he's there."

"You can't call now anyway," he says, and puts himself between the telephone and me.

And then I lose it.

"What right do you have to decide for me? I want to talk to my husband, and I'll do it whenever the hell I please!"

"No," he says. "Not here," and remains blocking the phone.

"Fuck you," I say, and turn away to leave. After a couple of steps, I lift my nightgown, squat down, pull down my panties, and pee on the floor. Then I leave him standing there with a pool on the linoleum, return to my room, and slam the door shut.

The next day, I reflect on my actions, and I begin to understand how easy it is to acquire behavioral problems. I'm not a troublemaker, but when I have my freedom snatched from me, it's easy to become desperate and use whatever means I have to protest.

Carl visits and brings the kids. I get to see them for an hour in the cafeteria. It's good to see them, but I'm happy when I can return to the ward. I'm tired, too tired to be with them. I begin to realize that I need to stay here. I'm in no shape to go home yet. The kids wake up five or six times every night, and I can't do that. I need to get some sleep, to have some peace.

I try to adapt to life on the ward. I feel closed in and do my best to tolerate it, but I need to feel a sense of freedom. I notice the smoking room. Before we had kids, I used to smoke at parties, and now I feel the urge to smoke again. I need to be able to make my own decisions, to be in control of something in my life. During the day, I'm allowed to take a walk with a staff member down to the grocery store. I buy cigarettes, light beer, cider, and snacks. I can't smoke without something to drink. Smoking and drinking used to go hand-in-hand for me. Back at the ward, I invite everyone to a party. I offer the other patients light beer and cider. The atmosphere is lighthearted, and we're having a great time until an attendant comes in and says we're not allowed to drink alcoholic beverages on the ward. It doesn't matter. I've started smoking again, and that in itself feels like a party. It's a little forbidden, and I'm acting defiant.

Daytime: I paint naïve pictures with symbols and love messages. I'm social and interact with the other patients. Soon, there's a whole gang sitting and drawing together. I organize an art exhibit and hang up our works in the corridor. In the day room, I hold a disco party and invite the others to dance. I'm full of energy, fun, and games.

When Carl or Mom visits, I always ask them to bring coffee cake and candy so I can share with the others. The staff think I'm disturbing the other patients. They're sad, and I am happy, happy and twittering with everyone. I have a newfound freedom, am creative and write poetry.

On the ward, all ages are represented. There's the silent teenage girl with the long hair. You hardly notice her; she takes up less room than a shadow. I give her my new, thin, silver-colored radio and headset. I got it from Carl, but I prefer my clumsy old one, where I can use the preset channels instead of tuning them in.

She carries it everywhere. Music can do wonders for a sad soul. Now it looks like she has a smile on her lips.

There's the woman who's going to be a grandmother. For her, a huge step on the stairway of life, a step down, closer to the end. Imagine, that such joyful news can make someone so sad.

There's the single mom with two kids who works in a clothing store. She can't make ends meet. There's never enough time, and the stress takes its toll. Her daughter usually tells her when it's time, time for her mom to stay on Ward 22 again.

"Mom, you've got a stress rash on your ear again. It's time to check in."

A few days on Ward 22 gives her a chance to catch her breath. She sleeps, eats, and winds down. The staff often recognize the new patients. They come in and out. I swear to myself that I will never come back here again.

In my room, there's a girl. She's tall and very thin, a walking skeleton covered in skin. Everyone can see that she's anorexic. Her bones protrude, and it hurts me to look at her. Most of the time, she's in bed. I think, isn't there any better care to be had? Will they let a young girl die, just like that?

We don't speak the same language. One day, I give her one of my drawings. The next day I receive one from her. Another day, there is a little candy on my pillow. It's from the thin girl who needs it more than anyone. I seldom see her in the cafeteria, and when she is there, she sits and pushes the food around her plate without eating. She never moves a morsel to her lips. Her friend is often there for visits. I don't know for sure if it's a girl or a boy. She has an androgynous appearance. Sometimes I see them lying on her bed in our room, as if the friend wants to shelter a brittle little baby bird.

There's Alice, big as a man, dressed in a suit and tie. Her hair sticks out in complete, uncombed disorder. If she didn't have such huge, floppy breasts, you would easily mistake her for a man. She smokes and swears like a sailor. She gets angry too, but I'm not afraid, I always have a retort. Then she snorts and continues smoking her cig. Sometimes she yells at me.

Some patients look like they just need a big hug. Leif, the overweight guy going through puberty, is soft and kind, but so lonely in all of life's trials. Fredrik, a father from the neighborhood, is convinced that his kids aren't his; his wife must have had an affair.

He's been on meds for a long time because of schizophrenia, and the medicine made him unable to have children, he believes. His wife and son come to see him, and I'm struck by the likeness between the son and Henrik. Later, we speak and I ask, "Why don't you have a DNA test instead of going around like this?"

"She doesn't know what I think," he says. "Then she'll think I'm even more paranoid. Her father is a psychiatrist. I have to be careful about what I say."

Alfred, a sly old man with shining light blue eyes, is old, but his soul is young. He spits, hisses, and smokes a pipe. He has such a dirty mouth that I blush whenever he speaks, but I get used to it after a while. He's fun, and we bicker some in the smoking room. Alfred is one of the old-timers on Ward 22. He comes and goes regularly, just like Alice.

There's a foreign man who wanders sadly up and down the corridor. I talk to him, and he tells me that he comes from Turkey. His beloved is still there, but he can never go back because of his political views. He has a broken heart. I make him a painting that symbolizes his unhappy love. He's moved. It's the nicest painting he's ever received.

It's a different world on Ward 22. So many different people with different fates. I approach and speak with some of them, but others are psychotic and impossible to reach.

There's an old woman who is psychotic, maybe suffering from an isolation psychosis after having been alone too long. She locks herself in the lavatory, stands, screams, and shouts in front of the mirror.

A middle-aged woman moves into our room. She is always naked and packs and unpacks her things all night long. One night, when she's at it again, I can't sleep, and have to move onto a mattress in a therapy room.

Then we have Peter. Peter and I become friends. We can laugh together amid all the sorrows. We sit in the smoking room, puffing away and making puns. Sometimes at midday, sometimes in the middle of the night. It's been a long time since I've had so much fun. He is a gambling addict and has almost gambled away his home and family. His wife is ready to leave him for good. He has spent all their money and then some on gambling. He's kind and funny, and we play pranks together. Well, it's mostly me playing pranks on him. Most of the others walk around in a depressing circle. I am now a west wind, moving around with energy and ingenuity. I talk with everyone and get this one or that one involved in small projects. I read poems by Nils Ferlin, paint a lot, write my own poems and letters to my near and dear. In the letter to my sister-in-law, I thank her for supporting Carl. She works in our company and has greater responsibility now that Carl has to be at home with the kids. I write another letter to an old friend who is no longer my friend. We saw a lot of each other but had a fight and lost touch.

I write a book for my kids about Jenny Penguin and Carl the Bear. A little tale with short texts and pictures about how we met, married, and had children.

One day, I'm standing around talking to a ward attendant.

"Have you noticed how easy it is to see how the patients here are doing?" I ask him.

"No," he answers. "How do you mean?"

"The ones who are the worst off walk around in their nightshirts," I explain. "Those who feel somewhat better wear their bathrobes. The ones who feel okay put on their own clothes. If they feel even better than that, they care about how they look. Then they comb their hair, put on makeup, shave, and use perfume," I say.

He looks around the ward, where various patients are walking in the corridor.

"Yeah," he says, "you're probably right. I've never thought about it before."

Thought, I think to myself. *They haven't done much of that in psychiatry.*

I seldom walk around in hospital dress. I feel too healthy for that. When I wake up in the middle of the night, I sometimes go have a cig, and then I'll use the hospital bathrobe over my nightgown.

On Ward 22, everyone takes medication, no matter what his or her problem is. Many years ago, difficult cases were lobotomized, but now they've found a more cost-effective way, now they prescribe meds instead. Though I've heard about electric shock therapy still being administered. When will they start using more dramatic methods? The meds don't help me. I'm afraid of electric shocks, but what else can they use? It feels like I've landed in *One Flew Over the Cuckoo's Nest*. For the medicine to work, the patient must believe it will, but I don't.

When I had hyperthyroidism many years ago, the doctor said I had to take pills for at least a year and a half and maybe for the rest of my life. Every eight hours, lots of pills. I really hate medicines. I took the tablets for three months and then decided to stop. At that time, I was in Venezuela, so I couldn't go to my doctor and have tests, but I figured I would recognize the symptoms if they returned and then I would get help.

I had no symptoms and haven't had any since then, and that was seven years ago. For me, that's proof doctors can't always predict the outcome of meds. The pharmaceutical companies supply them with all the facts about them, and their motivation is to sell their products. Most of the meds are tested on mice and men. How are they ever going to know which medicines will help who, against what, and in what dose? It's an impossible puzzle to solve. Everyone is different.

Medicines are, however, a very useful tool for psychiatrists, since they have no other tools. Not here on Ward 22 anyway. I see different doctors, but there's one who takes primary responsibility for me, and that's Dr. K. Mr. Hot-shot Doctor, fancy-pants, wears new shirts every day and swaggers around in the corridor. I point out to him that he can iron them before he puts them on. They get so creased lying in their boxes. We're the same age, and I call him Dr. Flannel, because he wants to seem tough but is pretty soft, and it rhymes with his name. Other times I call him Mister Caramel, because he seems to think he's a fox, but Carl has faith in Dr. K and wants to trust him because there is no one else.

After I've been more than a week on Ward 22, Dr. K says to my husband, "The medicine doesn't seem to have an effect on your wife. She's getting the dose of a two-hundred-pound man who's six feet tall." (I am 5 feet 5 inches and weigh 110 pounds.)

It started with sedation, which put me to sleep for fourteen hours and led to gaps in my memory. Then they used neuroleptics, powerful antipsychotic drugs. The side effects are common and counteracted with other medicines, but all of this isn't mentioned much. Drugged people often can't speak up, and I understand why the doctors don't see any need for group therapy.

When the chemical doesn't have the desired effect, they increase the dose; when the increased dose doesn't do the trick, they change the medicine, and so on. Many kinds of medicines on the list of those I took: Nitrazepam, Stesolid, Zyprexa, Inderal, Nozinan, Theralen, Tegretol, Imovane.

I feel terrible. My speech is sloppy. My joints are stiff, and I walk like a robot. I don't recognize myself. My thoughts float away even more than they did before. When the phone rings, I run to answer it. I think it's my father to say he's coming to get me and take me away from here.

I don't get out of the ward often, but today I'm going to have lunch with my two sisters. It's liberating to get out into reality, the real world. I'm under the influence of drugs, and I feel strange. Are people watching me? Can they tell that I'm different, that I walk funny, don't feel like myself? However, no one seems to notice.

We have lunch at a restaurant in the city. It's late afternoon, too late for lunch and too early for dinner. It's quiet at the restaurant, and that suits me fine. We sit down at a table outside and order lunch. I have a beer and light up a cigarette. I draw in a deep breath. I feel free. It's been a long time since I went to a bar, had a beer, and smoked. Not since we had kids. It's liberating, and I feel free.

Eva, my sister, has recently begun dating her ex-boyfriend again. It's been over a year since they split up.

I know intuitively that she's pregnant, and I ask her, "Is there something you want to tell us?"

"No," she says. "What? What do you mean?"

"You know what I mean," I say.

"No, I don't know what you mean," she answers.

"Good news," I say.

"No, what are you talking about?"

"You're pregnant!" I say.

"No," she says. "Really, I'm not."

A few days later, she has a pregnancy test and it's positive. She's expecting! She didn't know it when we met, but I knew it. She's astonished.

Then she calls me.

"How did you know I was pregnant?"

"I don't know. I just knew."

That evening, I have a cigarette in the smoking room of Ward 22. The summer evening is lovely, and I press my nose against the tiny ventilation window to experience the cool, clean air. I write a poem to her.

A New Child

What does the sunset say?
A little boy or a little girl?
The sky shimmers in light blue and pink.
It's so lovely,
And the answer is:
It doesn't matter.

All newborns are beautiful!
So wonderful
So fine
So heavenly

The next day, I do a pastel drawing for a congratulations card. Outside I put a heart in light blue and pink. Inside I write out the poem for her.

One day when I'm standing at the window in the smoking room, watching, I see something remarkable. It's a father out bicycling with his son. Nothing strange about that, but the thing is the bike— I've never seen anything like it. The father has a regular bicycle, but attached to the baggage rack is another piece, a half bike with handlebars, and on it is a boy in his own seat with pedals, and he's pedaling away. It's not a tandem bike but a special kind of "trailer bike." I think, I must get one if Lucas doesn't learn to ride a bike. For children with autism, bike riding doesn't come easily. Coordinating balance, pedaling, and steering is an extremely difficult task.

Another day, they roll an obviously autistic man, around forty-five years old, into our ward. He can't speak but makes some sounds. It's so improbable to have a patient like that on our ward. How do they know if he's feeling bad psychologically? Has he shown any self-destructive behavior? Are just they moving him here and keeping him drugged so he'll forget what upset him in the first place?

I believe it must be a joke. Are they fooling me? Do they want to scare me out of my psychosis? I feel like a marionette in a puppet theater, where someone else is holding the strings, directing, and setting out props to suit my life and me. I have a hard time landing, finding my way back to reality. The medicines make me more confused; my ego is the middle of the universe, and I believe everything revolves around me.

My mom and sisters are allowed to come visit. We sit in the day room. They've brought my old photo albums. We sit and leaf through and rehash old memories. They do most of the talking, recalling various details from trips we've taken together.

When they've left, I begin to focus my thoughts inward. What do I want to do with my life? What do I want to do when I get out of here? For the past three years, I've been living in a bubble centered on the children. Carl has worked a lot and seldom been at home. I have taken on most of the responsibility for our kids. Initially, when Lucas was born, we still had a social circle, but in time, it shrank because we didn't have the energy or time to see our friends. The children, the business, and the house we were renovating took all of our time and energy. I've been living increasingly isolated in our little cocoon. It's as if I've ceased to exist. For years, I haven't done anything for myself. My life has been for the children, and the only thing I've cared about has been their welfare. Now I feel the need to develop myself.

I'm a chrysalis, ready to open into a butterfly. I want to test my wings, I want to fly, be free, and discover the world. I want to be someone, receive recognition, and re-conquer myself. I'm still hyperactive and have an enormous amount of energy and creativity. Nothing is impossible and the world lies at my feet. It's as if I'm young again.

I see ideas and potential everywhere.

In a gossip magazine, I read about Betty Bjurström, who died recently. She lived the life of an adventurer. When she was an artist in a revue at the China Theater in Stockholm, she made headlines with daring topless dances. Then she became a movie star and was lured to Italy by a director who actually wanted her to be his mistress, but in a bomb shelter in World War II, during an air raid, she met Renato Senise, whom she married. In Italy, she was unjustly accused of espionage and interrogated by Mussolini's secret police. The lead officer in the interrogation fell in love with her and proposed, and when she refused she was imprisoned. Renato's uncle, who was the police chief of Rome, had her freed. She had a stormy marriage with Renato that spanned several countries. (He was later arrested and imprisoned for espionage as well as economic crimes.) When their marriage fell apart and Renato refused to give her a divorce, he shot her in a fit of jealousy, which crippled her for life.

Renato was sentenced to a couple of months in a mental hospital, and Betty moved back to Sweden. For a while, she worked in a hair salon and ran a gift shop. For many years after that, she had a clothing shop in a chic part of central Stockholm. She continued to hobnob with the jet set and traveled the world over to attend glamorous parties. In the article, it says that her son, Vincent, is making a movie about her dramatic life. I believe I would fit the role of his mother perfectly, yes, when she was in her thirties and after. I immediately begin to write a letter to Vincent, telling him why I think I can do the role justice. I tell him about my life, full of joy and sorrow. I'm not particularly experienced as an actor except for school plays, but I don't think that will be much of a problem. I've experienced so much in real life that inspires me. I save the letter and think of adding a few photos of myself and then sending it when I get out of here.

In ten days, former president Bill Clinton is coming to Stockholm. He is going to speak at a leadership seminar at the Cirkus arena. The theme is "Business and Politics – Corporate Citizenship." It's the first time he'll have been in Sweden to speak in that context. The elite from the Swedish business and political world will be there to hear him.

Carl and I will of course be there, because our company, Talarforum, is organizing the event. The media hype is immense, and the newspapers print something every other day about Clinton's visit: what he gets paid, the kind of security that's needed, who is going to be there, and so on. It's an important event, and Carl has worked hard for over a year to make it happen. Afterwards, there will be a huge gala dinner, and I don't have anything to wear. . . . Creative powers engaged, I sketch and paint different dresses. My wedding dress was a perfect fit, so I begin with that model, adding and taking away. I ask the other patients for advice, what they think about this or that tailoring, the silk with a little tulle, maybe these colors? Everyone gets involved and thinks it's fun, while the caregivers laugh behind my back and think I'm imagining it all.

Carl visits me that afternoon. He's brought a copy of *Dagens Industri,* Sweden's daily business newspaper, and shows me the ad for the Clinton event. I think it's a bad job, which could have been done better. There are still a lot of seats left, and I feel it's important to market the event in an appropriate way. I discuss it with him, but he doesn't seem to listen. In our company, I work some with marketing and PR, and I want to help in developing a more innovative and effective advertisement. My creativity and self-confidence have no bounds, and I'm convinced I can create an ad that will be a prize-winner in the world of advertising. With enormous energy, I begin designing an exceptionally fantastic ad. My thoughts circle around basic values such as hope, faith, and charity, for these are emotions that are strong within me now.

I draw several sketches, and the next time Carl comes, I'm fired up and want to show him what I've done. He isn't interested and hardly looks. He's more concerned about me, worried that I'm still not sleeping as I should and that I have difficulties keeping calm.

I'm disappointed, since I've put my entire soul into producing something good and Carl doesn't seem to care. However, my self-confidence is at its zenith and I'm completely convinced that the ad will win an award if it's published.

"Don't you see? We can win a prize for this, and it'll sell the event. There are still seats left that need to be sold. Don't you see how great that would be?" I say.

Carl doesn't see. I must do something. I can't let a chance like this—winning a Golden Egg, the prize in a huge Swedish advertising contest—slip through my fingers. If Carl can't see it, I'll have to take the matter into my own hands, and I do.

From the telephone on the ward, I call *Svenska Dagbladet,* a large daily newspaper. I introduce myself and tell them that I want to have a full-page ad running for several days. I can't fax or email the copy, so I describe on the phone how it should look, what it will say, and which colors it needs. They understand how it's to be done and will make sure to develop a layout that will look exactly as I've intended. I feel terribly satisfied with myself.

Carl visits the day after. He is completely livid, almost beside himself with anger. He has received an order confirmation from the ad department at *Svenska Dagbladet* for a half million kronor (around $70,000), for an ad that will run for several days. I feel he's overreacting. He didn't even want to see my ads. I had told him that if he wasn't interested or felt he didn't have time, I'd have to fix it myself, but he obviously missed that part. Carl shouts at the doctors. How could they let this happen? Don't they have any control in this place? How lax is it? Don't they see what the patients are doing? Dr. K defends himself by saying that it's common for hyperactive people to begin spending and wasting a lot of money.

After that, I have stricter rules. They hope that having fewer stimuli will get me to slow down. No longer sharing with three others, I'm now isolated in a room of my own. I'm restricted to my room and may not be out on the ward, except when it's mealtime or when I have a cigarette. I'm permitted to smoke only once an hour, on the hour. I'm not allowed to use my radio, listen to music. I'm not allowed to have any newspapers or watch TV. The only things I can have in my room are a pen, paper, and a book. I'm not allowed to place or receive calls. I'm not allowed to have any contact with my mother or sisters. No one may visit me, except for Carl. The doctors and personnel say they're doing this for my own good. In my medical records, it says, "*They've tried to support the patient and help her not spread out verbally to other patients.*"

Carl doesn't want me to be isolated but has no means to counter the doctors' orders. Besides, he wants to believe that the doctor knows what he's doing. I try to adapt to solitude, but it feels unfair, like I'm being punished. The only joy I had was in being with the other patients. Now I have nothing. I still sleep for just a couple of hours every night, and the days and nights are endless.

I feel awful. The medicine makes me feel strange. My chest hurts. One morning, when I'm standing half-naked in front of the mirror in the bathroom, I pinch my nipple and a little milk oozes out. It has been more than six months since I stopped nursing. Am I pregnant? Or is it because I long for my kids? Is that why it's happening?

I know what it was like when the kids were small and I was nursing. If they weren't close by and I missed them, or even just thought about them, my breasts would begin to lactate. My body has a mind of its own sometimes and expresses what my soul would—its longing. I have an IUD. The risk of pregnancy is minimal. But there is always a margin for error. When did I have my last period? I don't have one now, since my IUD releases hormones. How will I know if I'm pregnant? Imagine if I'm expecting! It's not possible, not now. How would we manage another child? It would never work. We'd die. And think of all those medicines? God, what kind of damage could they do to a little embryo? I've read in magazines that neuroleptics and other strong sleeping pills can cause brain damage. It usually says that when giving these medicines to pregnant women, one must weigh the risks against the advantages. Pregnant women do actually take the stuff, but what advantages can outweigh that risk? Can you ever defend causing brain damage to your child?

I can't take any more upheaval in my life right now, but still, a little baby, a miracle, how could you say no to that? Maybe a child would be good? Let us get back on our feet. Become whole as a family. I ask to have a pregnancy test. They don't question me, and I supply a urine sample. The results are negative. I'm relieved not to be forced into making a difficult decision.

Nozinan is medicine I take every day here. It's a neuroleptic that is used to treat schizophrenia, the manic phases of bipolar disorder, and certain other psychotic behaviors. Common side effects are dizziness, fatigue, shakiness, stiffness, and cramping or shakes in the fingers and hands. In some cases, there may be a particular form of inner restlessness, which manifests itself in difficulty in sitting still. Large doses can cause facial tics, grimacing, and strange tongue movements. Low blood pressure and heart palpitations can occur, increasing the risk of fainting. Less common side effects are worsening of visual focus, difficulty in reading small print, enlarged breast glands in men, and secretion of milk in women.

Another drug I'm being given is Zyprexa. Common side effects are anxiety, involuntary motor disturbances, shakes, and muscle stiffness or spasms and speech impairment. In rare cases, after long use, women can experience milk secretion from the breasts or missing or late menstruation.

The same day that I express my worry about being pregnant, the doctor quits giving Zyprexa. Instead, I receive Tegretol. It belongs to a group of drugs called anti-seizure medications. It works by stopping the diffusion of the signals in the brain that would cause an epileptic attack. Common side effects are vomiting, nausea, dizziness, uncoordinated muscle movement, and fatigue. The next morning, I vomit after taking my meds. The same happens after another couple of days. Following my first days in isolation, the doctor feels I've calmed down, and he tells me they can decrease my meds, since I've vomited.

Carl is not so sure, however. He thinks I've seemed better and doesn't want to risk a regression. He wants me to be able to sleep, so I'll get better faster and come back home. Because of that, the doctor decides instead to spread the same dose out over the course of the day, that way decreasing the amount I take each time. When I hear this, I get angry. I feel powerless and want to leave.

"Isn't there any other place where I can get treatment?" I plead with Carl. "I don't want to have to take meds that make me sick."

"Eva was supposed to check it out, but it seems she hasn't found anything yet. I think you'll have to stay here for the time being. I think you've gotten better. I promise to call Eva again."

"No f—ing way I've gotten better. I feel terrible. You don't understand what it's like, being locked into a damned room and being drugged. I don't recognize myself. I can't think clearly. I can't talk, I walk funny. Soon, I'll do the same as the others."

"What?" Carl asks. "What do you mean?"

"They hide their meds under their tongue and spit them out when the staff isn't looking."

The next day I have a talk with the doctor. Carl has spoken with him, and I'm suddenly being accused of having put my fingers down my throat and vomiting up the meds on purpose. That's not true. My body has quite simply had enough of this punishment, but Dr. K doesn't believe it.

"We have to discuss other solutions, since you won't cooperate with the medication," Dr. K says to me. "We have treated you for over two weeks and haven't gotten the results we hoped for. You're still in overdrive and not sleeping as you should."

I suggest aspirin, Ibuprofen, or Advil. The doctor purses his lips. That wasn't exactly what he had in mind. A chill runs down my spine, and I'm afraid he's thinking it's time for electric shocks. I didn't think things could get or feel any worse, but here we are.

"We could try giving you an injection that will stay in your system and work over time. Another alternative is lithium, a pharmaceutical that's proven and has been in use for a long time," says Dr. K. When he's finished, I turn around and walk out the door, leaving him standing alone in the room.

Stuff me full of meds—how will that solve my problems? I think. I will definitely become chronically ill if I stay in this place. If they continue to drug me like this, I'll never get well.

He calls for me to return, but I just leave, get away from there. When I don't come back, he has the attendants fetch me. They say the doctor has decided to give me an injection. They try to bring me back to the room. I refuse, run away, and resist. They fail to get me to come, and finally they send the largest of the attendants. Behind him, there are at least five others. He's enormous. Probably six foot two or more, with a big belly and streaks of gray in his hair. He homes in on me. He's unstoppable, and I don't stand a chance. He picks me up as if I were Jane and he's King Kong and carries me over his shoulder to the examination room. I kick, scream, and fight.

"I DON'T WANT ANY MORE MEDICINE!"

He carries me in, and they wrestle me down on the table and hold me there. Terrified, I lie on my back with the attendants everywhere around me, holding my arms and legs. My pulse is about two hundred and my heart hurts. I am afraid I'll have a heart attack. I can see them giving me a shot to make me sleep and then my heart stops and I die. A few days earlier, before I was isolated in my room, I read an article about heart attacks. It's been said that, if you have cardiac arrest, you have only a few minutes to react before it's too late and you die. When I've gone to sleep, the staff will all leave me. I'll have cardiac arrest, and no one will be at my side to give me the emergency treatment I need. *I'm going to die!*

I have a panic attack.

"I want Carl here. I want to call my husband. I want Carl to be here if you're going to give me a shot," I say.

If Carl were here, he would stay by my side. He would never let me die, never, I think.

"Okay," says Dr. K. "You get one call."

The attendants let go of my arms, and Dr. K gives me his cell phone so I can make the call. I punch the number to the office. I ask for Carl, but the woman who answers says that Carl isn't there.

"Try his cell instead," she says. In a feverish rush, I try his cell number, but all I get on the other end is his very businesslike voicemail.

"Can't you get a hold of him?" says the doctor.

"One more try," I beg, and Dr. K looks at his watch. He doesn't have time to answer.

I try our home phone number and hope to God that Carl will answer.

"Hey, you've reached the family of . . ." Voicemail there too.

"Carl, if you can hear me, answer. I need you now. They're going to give me a shot and I don't want to—"

"We can't wait any longer," says Dr. K, and he takes the phone from my grip. "I'm going away for the weekend, and I have a plane to catch."

The nurse has already prepped the injection. I'm in total panic. Tears are streaming down. They turn me violently on my stomach, pull down my pants and stick the needle in my buttock. It stings a little, and then they let me go. The attendants disperse, and the doctor hurries off so he doesn't miss his plane.

"I'm still awake," I say to the nurse who hasn't left my side.

"Yes," she says. "Why wouldn't you be?"

"I thought the shot would make me sleep," I say.

"No, you'll stay awake the whole time."

No one had told me what to expect. I thought I would be put to sleep.

I don't die, but it's far from over. Now I have a drug in my body, a deposit of Cisordinol-Acutard, yet another neuroleptic, this one with a long-lasting effect. It works for three days and is used to treat serious psychoses, manic attacks, and relapses of chronic psychosis. Just the knowledge that I have a medication inside me that will be there over a longer period gives me a claustrophobic feeling. Relatively soon after the shot, I suffer a terrible side effect, akathisia, which means I have an uncomfortable prickly sensation all over. My skin is crawling, and I wish I could jump out of my body. I want to check out and turn the room key over to someone else. I can't sit still. I can't relax. It's impossible to do anything, and I need to be in constant motion. I walk, walk, and want to escape from myself, but my body follows along, and the uncomfortable sensation continues.

No one seems to cares about the side effects. Akathisia is an indication that the dose is too high. The most important corrective step is to decrease the dosage, but they can't do that because it's already stored in my body.

My body won't tolerate more neuroleptics. However, since Dr. K has no other tools than drugs, he has insisted on continuing to try new ones. The only good thing is that Tegretol, which has vomiting as a side effect, has been struck from my list of medicines. I had plenty of problems of my own before, which is why I ended up on Ward 22. The meds just make it doubly difficult to cope with them.

There's no time to deal with my own sorrow and anxiety. Instead, I have to deal with the side effects. The meds are only worsening my condition, and I feel powerless. Suspecting that medication is the wrong track, I'm beginning to lose faith that I'll ever recover.

The whole weekend is hell. Fortunately, though, the worst of the akathisia wears off after the first twenty-four hours.

I'm angry and upset and ask to speak with the psychologist, with my husband present. The forced injection is the worst experience of my life. I was afraid I'd die. It was an assault and felt like a rape.

There's a bulletin board in the corridor. A small notice is posted on it: HAVE YOU BEEN GIVEN THE WRONG TREATMENT? YOU CAN TURN TO THE PATIENTS' ADVISORY COMMITTEE. I take one of the brochures and contemplate whether to report them immediately, but decide to let it rest. Who the hell is going to believe someone who has been committed to a mental ward? I figure there'll probably be a better occasion. Carl and I meet the psychologist, and I tell her about the injection episode. I say that I want to report the doctor to the Patients' Advisory Committee. She listens, doesn't say much.

THE SPIRIT OF HEALING

I'm looking for my own ways to heal. I understand that it's my journey, which I must make alone. I have no idea how long it will take or which way to go, but I'm sure I'll understand, once I'm there. The meds are no good; on the contrary, they only make the journey longer. They take me on paths that get me lost and lead me in circles.

I continue to search for answers concerning my father. Is Father a secret agent, or is he perhaps a member of some secret research project about genetically manipulated humans? Maybe I have a clone somewhere, who's living with him in South America. Her name is June. All this is very confidential—state secrets of the highest level—and that's why he can't come see me.

I'm not allowed to answer the phone in the corridor anymore, since I'm in isolation, but I usually stick my head out to hear if it's for me, if it could be my dad.

I meet a new patient in the smoking room. She bears a striking resemblance to my deceased grandmother, as I remember her from when I was little. Even her hoarse, smoky voice reminds me of my grandmother. That same night, I wake up at around three. I lie completely still in bed and hear a heartbeat: thud, thud, thud, thud. I understand that it's my grandmother's heart beating. The room vibrates with heartbeats. I hear them quite clearly. Then it's quiet, and she's gone. Finally, she'll have peace, now that she understands I know what's going on with her son, my father. She has always known that he was an agent but has never been able to tell us. She took the secret with her to her grave when she died many years ago. Now she can finally let go, and I feel how her soul, which has remained here, disappears far away up in the air and out of the room, when the heartbeat ceases.

On waking the next morning, I'm dazed. The experience was intense and so real that it felt like the truth, but I understand that I mustn't utter a word of these thoughts to anyone. They won't let me out of here if I do. Later, I find out that antipsychotics can have side effects such as hallucinations, intense dreams, nightmares, and an altered sense of reality.

I've asked Carl countless times if there's an alternative to Ward 22. There must be a private clinic somewhere. I understand that I need treatment and rest and that I can't come home yet, but there must be somewhere other than this terrible place, where all they do is keep the patients drugged and wait until they give in. If I wasn't crazy before I was admitted, I'll certainly go crazy in here. What I don't know is that I've been committed. And Carl can't actually do anything about it.

Soon, my body will adjust to the drugs and want more. I've been here now for more than two weeks, and I see the poor patients that come and go on the ward and who constantly come back for more medication. They've learned to handle life with the help of them and can't manage without.

I want to go to a calm and peaceful place, where I can just exist. I want to be taken care of, I want to have someone to talk to who'll listen and take the time, and I want to be fussed over, have massages, and work out. A place where both body and soul can have some space. A place that gives me peace and quiet, where I can rest and build up my self again, without medicines.

I do everything possible to work on the feelings of grief and exhilaration that my psychosis and the meds bring out in me. Before they locked me in my room, I could throw my energy into lots of paintings and poems. Now I'm allotted only one piece of paper a day. Luckily, I find an old copy of *Science Illustrated* in my room, and in the margins I write how I feel and other thoughts. Before, I had my own radio with earphones, and I danced to music. To keep some kind of balance, I meditate and do yoga and stretching exercises. I stand on my head in bed and let the blood run down until I'm completely dizzy. I sit on the floor, bend double like a jackknife, hold my toes, and press my stomach to my legs. This stretches the backs of my thighs nicely. Then I sit in the lotus position, relax, and let my world fly away.

Sometimes, I lie on my bed, with my feet on the pillow, like Pippi Longstocking, and think. Damn it! I'm sure as hell going to get through this. I'm strong and nothing will break me. When it's sunny, I move the furniture around my room and push the bed over to the window. I lie there and let the May sun shine down on me. Its warmth is wonderful on my skin, and it supplies me with energy.

"You're very tanned," say the staff.

"Yes, you can sunbathe behind glass," I say. "Didn't know that, did you?"

Other days, I go to the shower and have a mini-spa. Slowly, slowly, I turn up the thermostat to maximum. I sit on the floor, lean against the wall; the water splashes my face, breasts, stomach, and legs. I sit there for a long time, letting the water wash over me. The steam builds up, like a fog, filling the entire bathroom. After a while, there's a knock on the door.

"Will you be ready soon?" says the attendant outside.

"I'm in the shower. I'm not finished yet."

"There are others waiting," he says.

"Well, let them wait then. They're not going anywhere," I say and giggle to myself.

"Well, all right, a little while longer," he says.

I continue to shower, letting the water bounce off my body and enjoying the humidity. Knock, knock. A little harder this time.

"Now you've been in there a half hour. That's enough," he says.

"Finished in a sec," I call, to appease him, so he'll go away, but I don't move a muscle. I just sit. The warmth spreads throughout my body and makes it pliable and relaxed. I exist in the moment. After a while, the door jerks open and the attendant sticks in his head.

"What are you doing in here?"

"What the hell? You damned pervert!" I yell as loudly as possible. "Get out of here! Is there nowhere I can be left alone?" I scream to embarrass him. He shrinks back and goes away.

Conversation with Dr. K:

"How are you doing in your room?" he asks.

I'm still isolated and not allowed out on the ward.

"Fucking awful. There's nothing to do. I can't talk to anyone, and I feel terrible from all the medicines. I'd like to stop taking them now."

"You're still in high gear and need to sleep, so I'm afraid that's not possible," says Dr. K.

"Carl's going to find another place and then I'll move out of here."

"I see. Well, that'll have to be later, not now anyway," he says.

"Oh no, why not?" I ask.

"You're here for compulsory care. You're not allowed to go anywhere."

"How long is the compulsory care?"

"Well, I decide that. It depends on how cooperative you are," he says, and his lips curve into a smile.

I feel myself turning cold and the color leaving my face. The dream of getting out of here is gone.

Back in my room, I lie down in bed and drift off. When I wake, it's past five o'clock and I realize I'll be late for dinner.

When I arrive in the day room, everyone is seated. The only open spot is next to Karlsson with the gray hair and hunchback. What bad luck, I think to myself. It's such a chore to talk to him, 'cause he just rambles on and on about taxes, business, and that they stole his company, which was worth *so* much. I serve myself food from the cart and sit beside him. He starts talking immediately. I try to listen to what he says and answer as well as possible, but he doesn't hear my answers. After a while, I give up. Some people are difficult to talk to. I talk the ears off people, but they think it's fun and they laugh, flocking around me and wanting to get in on it. I feel like Jesus, leading my apostles. My word is law, which they blindly and faithfully obey. It's an awesome feeling.

Karlsson, on the other hand, is no fun, and we take long detours to avoid him. If we meet him in the corridor, we dive into the restroom to avoid getting mired in his grinding litany going around and around with no end. I leave Karlsson and try to see if there's anyone I can talk to. At my table, there are only new faces today. The group of people I know is at the other table. Across from me is an old woman. She looks trim and proper. Her white hair is well groomed, and she's wearing street clothes, not the hospital robe that some others wear. Her hands are shaking, and she has difficulty getting anything on her fork. I see her struggle, but everything falls off and she doesn't get anything in her mouth, no matter how hard she tries. I go out into the kitchen and ask for a soupspoon. I go to my seat again and give her the spoon. She gives me a grateful look and takes it from me. I think, *Where are the attendants? They're so deplorable—never see what the patients need!*

Outside the smoking room window, there's often a little bird that sits on the sill. I usually stand and watch it from the inside. He gives me hope that one day I'll be able to fly away, free, just like him, wherever I want. One morning, I'm in the smoking room, alone with some of the staff.

"Have you seen my buddy?" I ask and point out into the air.

The bird is gone, so they don't see it.

"So you've got another invisible friend, besides your father?" one of them asks.

I purse my lips, being used to their jokes, and can strike back hard.

"No, it's real," I answer and walk over to the window, standing there. After a little while, the bird flies up and sits on the windowsill.

He flips his tail up and down some. His eyes meet mine for a second. I turn around and stare at the attendants in the room. They fidget, look embarrassed. Then they get up and leave.

"She's a real piece of work, that one," I hear one of them say on the way out.

José, one of the staff members, is friendly and likes to talk with me. He's the one who goes with me to the kiosk to buy cigarettes. He gives me extra crayons to draw with sometimes and brings me paper if I've filled my whole page. He knocks on my door.

"Hey, whatcha doin'?" he asks.

"Putting up my pictures."

The whole wall is full of drawings.

"Let's see," he says. "Nice! What is it?"

"The beginning of the universe," I answer and begin to explain. "Here's the birth of the sun, the stars, and the moon."

José tells me he's half Indian. He comes from a village high up in the mountains of Peru.

"We believe in other gods than you do here in Sweden," he says.

He starts to tell stories that his grandmother told him when he was little, about their beliefs.

Later, in the afternoon, I'm sitting alone in the smoking room and wondering: What happens when you die? Where do you go? Maybe the soul just moves on to new places. Are you born into another person or an animal, or is the soul transformed into some other matter?

I stand by the window and look out over the parking lot and the woods beyond. It's windy, and the treetops sway back and forth. High up in the sky, the clouds are rushing by.

Maybe you're just admitted to the universe when you die, into another context. Maybe the wind out there is a soul. I imagine that it's my dad's turn to be the wind. It's almost stormy out there. The wind increases, and I think it's my father, coming to say goodbye. The wind makes the walls creak, more like an autumn storm than a fresh spring breeze. There is a huge crescendo, and then all is calm and completely silent. I sit down on a chair facing the window. I close my eyes and sit still, lost in a trance, forgetting time and place.

I've never felt so relaxed, so free of tension in every single part of my body. My whole self is drawn to the floor, as if the earth's gravity has doubled. It's a peaceful feeling. After a while, I open my eyes. I look at my cigarette. The ash has grown long and fallen to the floor. I take a couple of deep drags and feel the nicotine intoxicate my brain. I've just finished and am ready to put it out, when something unusual captures my eye. A yellow nicotine spot forms on the filter when you smoke. It's usually round, but it's not now—it's shaped like a star. A yellow star. A completely distinct star. I'm surprised, in wonder, captivated. A star, how could it be a star?

I draw and write notes about things I experience, so as not to forget them in the chemical fog of medication. Back in my room, I do a pencil sketch of my hand with the star-spotted cigarette between my fingers.

I know that my father has left me forever, and I write a letter. A farewell letter. I give it to Esperanta, the wonderful Chilean woman in her fifties. She promises to take care of it for me. *Thank you, my angel. My guardian angel here, among the others*, I think.

She catches, receives and affirms, instead of rejecting, ignoring, or laughing off the wishes of a confused woman. She takes me seriously and treats me with warmth and respect, and I love her for it.

She hugs me, and warmth streams from her tiny body. I cry and don't want to let go of her. After a while, she frees herself. She looks at me with sorrow in her gaze and slowly caresses my cheek. I see that she knows what it's like to lose someone you love.

Angel and Esperanta, both from South America, are assigned as my special caretakers, and they've been with me to some of my doctor's and psychologist's appointments. They have heard me tell my story. They know it. Everyone here is either for or against, but I feel that Angel and Esperanta are on my side. They take me seriously but tell me to get my act together when I get out of hand. I listen then and am like a little girl scolded by her parents. How would I manage life on Ward 22 without them?

Most of the other attendants are just here to do their job as painlessly as possible. They sit in the corridor and read a magazine or sit in the smoking room smoking, waiting for the hours to tick away.

"Are you here again?" I tell the lazybones who don't give a damn about their jobs when I meet them in the smoking room. That shames them, and they lumber out with their tails between their legs. Others may laugh and give me a smart-alecky answer. "We need to keep an eye on you and check up on what you're doing," they say.

"But you don't need to smoke all the time," I say.

"No, but we might as well."

Sometimes, aggressive patients get involved, and the discussion heats up.

"Wait a minute, now it's getting too agitated in here," the attendants say then. "Time to break it up. If you've finished your cig, you have to leave."

I enjoy hearing them try to wiggle out of sticky situations.

Other times when I'm in the smoking room, I count out loud how many there are of each kind.

"One, two three four . . . uh oh, now there are more attendants than patients in here. Isn't there supposed to be a certain number of attendants on the ward checking on the patients? This is actually a psych ward. Security is of the utmost importance. Someone could commit suicide, and you wouldn't notice a thing."

That usually produces nervous laughter and embarrassment among the attendants, while the patients laugh their heads off.

"More! More!" Alfred cries and the others join in.

"You have the gift of the gab, don't you?" he says to me one day.

"Yeah, 'cept I can't answer back as well as you."

"No, you're right about that. I'll have to give you lessons," he says.

"Yeah, sure. Nice pipe you've got there. How's it taste?" I ask him.

"Mm, a lot better than that shit you smoke. This is pure tobacco, not that mixed shit. Here, wanna try?" he sends his slender black pipe over to me.

"How do I do it?"

"Just take a little puff."

I try it and have a puff.

"That's it, so, whaddaya say?"

"Not so bad."

"'Not so bad,' the hell you say! This is the best tobacco you can buy. Mild, and soft, like a girl's behind," he says and smiles his roguish smile. I like Alfred. He's real. Honest, uncomplicated, and kind through and through.

I've hung all my pictures of the creation of the earth and our family on my wall. They fill the whole wall and are placed in a special order, creating a cross. I count the drawings—there are nineteen in all. I write down names of the people in our immediate family. Then I count how many there are: one, two, three, four . . . If I include the unborn baby that my sister Eva is carrying, that makes nineteen people, the same number as the drawings I've done. It's all one in the larger context. You just have to find the connections to be able to see the big picture. I stand, pondering over my masterpiece. It's an impressive collection of drawings. In the middle, you can see the Big Bang, the sun, moon, planets, stars, then comes land and sea, people, sorrow, and joy.

STARTING TO RECOVER

Carl and I discuss future alternatives with the doctor and psychologist on the ward. What will happen when I'm released? There is a non-institutional care alternative, Sorteria, that I can visit. I think it sounds good, better than being here—maybe I can stop taking the meds then. I imagine that Sorteria can be a place for me to catch my breath, to visit when I need to get away or to sleep away a night or two when I need rest.

The kids wake up several times a night. Lucas woke up every forty-five minutes for several years. It's gotten better now, but he still wakes up four or five times and, so far, he's never slept through a whole night in his life. He's an early bird and wakes at 5:00 a.m., despite the fact that he goes to bed at 9:00. Sara also wakes up a couple of times nightly. Before, I dealt with the kids at night, but now I'm not sure how that will work, because I'm tired, way too tired to manage.

Later, I learn that Sorteria is open only during daytime, not at night, and it doesn't feel all that great anymore. Up till now, our division of labor has been I've taken on responsibility for the kids and Carl has taken on the business. We both agreed that was the best solution. Because of that, Carl isn't as close to them and can't console them the same way that I can. My only way to manage day-to-day at home will be if the kids can feel safe with Carl, if they can turn to him, instead of me.

I begin to realize that I must stay here at least long enough for Carl to build his relationship with our children. He needs time, lots of time, to bond with them, but I'm afraid my mother-in-law will take my place instead of giving Carl a chance to get closer to our kids. I know that she does it out of love and kindness, but I also know that Carl gladly lets her take over the responsibility because he's so unsure of his parental role. Each time I speak with Carl, I ask him how the kids are doing and what they're doing, and I express clearly my wish that he take responsibility for them and not ask my mother-in-law to help too much.

From the medical records:
Husband Carl describes feeling frustrated and beginning to feel more irritated by the patient, whom he experiences as partially hostile to treatment and cure. The undersigned [Dr. K] confirms the interpretation, meaning that there are probably psychological components in the patient that make her try to maintain her upset defensiveness.

So I don't lose hope, I keep my mind busy thinking about what I want to do when I get out of here. My thoughts go to my children and family. Soon it'll be summer and vacation time. I want us to be together and to do something as a family, just the four of us. I have an idea that we can rent an RV and drive around on our vacation. Then we'll be close. We can go to different places and stay where we please. We can sleep in the RV. It would be cozy, and I think the kids would like it. It would be like living in a cabin for them. We could bring a couple of bikes with kid seats and go on outings.

I think about the various holidays we celebrate. We usually celebrate Christmas at home. At Midsummer, we're usually in Dalarna with my mother and Ingvar. Maybe we could start a new tradition? What would the kids like? I happen to think of Halloween. That's truly a children's holiday. We can have a yearly Halloween dinner, where all the kids can dress up. I plan in detail how it will be, what games we'll play, what we'll eat, how we'll decorate the house.

I also think about my own future. What will I do afterwards? My husband and I have a business. I've been at home with the kids for a long time, and soon I'll go back to work. I'm not sure if it's a good idea to continue working together. I think I can start my own company and freelance instead. I don't know exactly what I'll do yet, but it'll come to me. I have a ton of ideas. Mainly, it's about new TV shows that I think I could develop and license. On the ward, at the dinner table, I brainstorm company names with the other patients. I believe it would be good to have some well-known people on the board, and that's how we coin the name, Starboard, and I design a logo with the name on it.

I also make drawings, with my family and love in the center. In one picture, a rainbow reaches down from the sky, down into a treasure chest full of money. It symbolizes that the treasures in life are my kids and my husband. Another depicts a heart, with the text "*el idioma unica*"—the only language, is love. A third shows a rainbow-colored boat with four candles. It symbolizes hope, and hope can only exist if we can be together, the four of us in our family.

I do everything I can to try to tolerate the isolation and find ways to manage, but it's not easy. I still have a lot of energy and it's difficult to be alone, without anyone to talk to. Carl comes by every day, and we talk on the phone too, but it's still very lonely. The days and nights contain many, many hours.

In the smoking room, it's possible for me to see the other patients and speak with them, but my time is limited to one cigarette, once an hour, and when I'm finished, I have to return to my room. I do everything I can to stay a little longer and, sometimes, by trickery, I can eke out another cigarette. Patients treat me to them on the sly, and other times I take one of the attendants' half-smoked cigarettes that they've saved for later and carefully hidden, though not well enough.

One day, I'm sitting in the smoking room when Amy, one of the attendants, sticks her head in.

"Are you still here?"

"Yes, I'm not finished yet," I say and show her my cigarette.

"I sat here smoking with you fifteen minutes ago," she says.

"No, that was yesterday," I say confidently.

All days are the same here. How would she know?

"No way, it was not. It was just now," she says and looks at the clock. "You must've had another one. You know the rules. One cigarette every hour on the hour. Now you won't get one at three o'clock, since you already had two."

Then she slams the door and leaves.

Amy makes me feel like a dog on a very short leash. I have no freedom and can't do what I want. If I try anything, she pulls a little harder, and I feel the collar tighten. I rise on my back paws and have difficulty breathing. Instead of loosening her grip, she takes in the slack. Less leeway for me. She curtails the only thing that gives me freedom: space, room to breathe, joy in life. She doesn't understand that she is slowly but surely breaking me down. She's leaving me nothing. She thinks she's doing what's best. That in her own way she's doing a good job.

But for me, it sucks.

Yet, in spite of everything, I like Amy. She means well. Beneath the hard surface, there's a kind heart. She's tall and thin, looks careworn, but tries to look fresh and youthful. You can tell by the lines around her mouth that she smokes. I ask if she has kids.

"Yes, a teenage boy."

"Are you single?"

"Yes," she says, "and a full-time mom."

I understand a little better why she is the way she is. She's used to being tough and hard but fair, in her opinion. I do everything possible to change her rules. What else can I do to survive here?

When Amy takes something away from you, there are others among the staff who will do the opposite. They have kind hearts. I feel such warmth coming mainly from the ones from South America. I speak Spanish with them, and we enjoy each other's company. What empathy—it shines in their eyes and through their actions! Sometimes, I receive an extra piece of paper or a colorful crayon, while the Swedes are dutiful and feel obliged to treat everyone equally, according to the rules. The cultural differences are very clear on Ward 22.

Today is Sunday, and I wake at six. I want to go to the Sweet Bun Church, the church for homeless people in a house in the Old Town. Every Sunday, they have a religious service and serve a free breakfast afterwards. My mother has helped out there for a couple of years. She usually arrives an hour before service and makes coffee and sandwiches. Many homeless people come there for the company but also to get a meal. Everyone is free to participate in his or her own way. Mom has told me how the homeless people usually get up and read a poem, sing a song, play the harmonica or whistle a tune. Some want to pray for someone they know is having a hard time. At Christmas, they have a beautiful crèche. My mother, who's a teacher, usually brings students to see it.

I'd like to go there and participate. Maybe it's my mental state, the many down-and-out people on my ward, or a longing for my mother that brings the church to mind. I don't know. I ask the caretakers and tell them I'd like to go there and listen to the service.

"No, that's not allowed," they answer. "Go back to your room. Stay there. You're going nowhere."

They don't know how it feels to be stripped of your freedom, not allowed to do as you please, not able to speak to those who mean the most to you. But I do know, and soon I won't be able to take it any longer.

After eight days in isolation, I've had enough. What have I done to deserve this punishment? I start feeling angry. I've given in long enough. I want out of here. I want to leave Ward 22. I want to see my mother, my sisters, and others who care about me.

In the evening, I yell at the personnel and defy them in any way I can. I refuse food, smoke more often than I'm allowed, sneak out into the corridor and try to call home, stay awake as long as I can, and refuse to go to bed. At 1:30 a.m., I ask for a shower. When I come out of the shower, they tell me to be quiet.

"I'm allowed to shower whenever the hell I want," I say.

"No, not if you disturb the other patients."

"It doesn't say anything about that in my rules."

"Be quiet now, so you don't wake the others. Go to your room."

I go to my room, but I don't want to stay there. I look around for another excuse to leave it. I take my water glass and walk back out into the corridor toward the bathroom to get some water. I meet the attendant.

"Are you out here again? You're supposed to be in your room."

"I only need a little water," I say and walk into the bathroom.

The attendant follows me. He's had enough of my shenanigans.

"That's enough. You know the rules. Into your room!" he screams.

I go ballistic. Tired of following orders, of being locked in my room, I'm holding a glass of water in my hand. I hold it up and throw it as hard as I can to the floor. The Duralex glass shatters into a thousand pieces, and water splashes all over.

"All right! You'll have to clean it up yourself," says the attendant.

He gets a broom and mop and forces me to wipe it up. Then he moves me forcibly to my room and closes the door after me.

"Now stay there and don't come out till tomorrow morning."

I stand by the window and look out.

Can't somebody take me away from here? Mom, where are you? I want to talk to you. To come over to your place and stay, be taken care of, and rest up. Please take care of me. I'm never getting out of here. Is no one listening? Is there no one out there who can help me?

It's the middle of the night and still quite dark outside.

I go to the light switch by the door.

I turn the ceiling light on and off, three short blinks, three long ones, three short ones: SOS.

Then I stand by the window, lean my forehead against the cold glass and look out into the black of night—but no one answers.

I turn the light on and off repeatedly, while tears stream down my face. I'm losing my will to live. It's running out, and soon there'll be nothing left. After a while, I lie on the bed and fall asleep in despair, exhausted.

Next morning, I apologize to the night staff. They're usually super nice, and I have no quarrel with them. I explain that I can't stand it any longer, being isolated like this, and that's why I'm so pissed off. A little later, the doctor confronts me about the previous night's rowdiness. He says this treatment has been arranged for my sake, so that I can calm down and have a chance to rest.

"I just want to see my mother," I answer.

"No," he replies. "You are not allowed to in your condition. We'll be treating you with Lithium now. Hopefully, that'll help you."

"Don't you get it? How many times do I have to tell you? I don't want more medicine!" I scream.

"If you don't calm down, we'll give you another injection," says Dr. K.

In horror, I recall the shot I was given a week earlier. I'll never submit to that again. But what can I do to resist? Nothing. The last time they gave it to me, they restrained me and they'll certainly do it again if I refuse—and all for my own good. I know perfectly well what would really have been for my own good: a private clinic without medications, with conversational therapy and comfortable massage treatments and spas, things that eliminate tension and provide peace of mind. But I know that will never happen.

It's Saturday evening, just past seven o'clock and time for evening snacks.

I go to the day room. The others have begun to gather around the sandwich cart in the middle of the room. I'm in no hurry. On the contrary, I want to stay as long as possible. I'm often the first to arrive and the last to leave, all in order to steal some extra minutes to be together with the others. I move in slow motion. I take a piece of wholegrain bread and apply the spread meticulously. I slowly slice a couple of pieces of cheese and put them on it. I make a cup of Earl Grey tea and sit down on the right-hand side of the table, to see the TV. I listen distractedly to the other patients and watch TV while I eat.

When the others have finished, they disappear. The ones who feel sociable sit with the staff on the couch. The others go have a smoke or head to their rooms. I have another sandwich, another cup of tea. Now I'm alone at the table. I enjoy being there, but I speak with no one, because I want to be invisible like a fly on the wall. Otherwise, I know they'll tell me to go to my room. I sit with my tea, and, when it's finished, I get a cup of hot chocolate.

The Bingo Lotto begins on TV. Patients and staff sit together on the sofa and play. It looks like fun. I'm still at the table, sipping my chocolate. They tabulate the row of numbers. Before they announce a number, I visualize it in my head. Imagine if I'd been allowed to play—I'd get them all right. I linger in this atmosphere of community until an attendant remembers his duty and jerks away from watching the TV.

"What are you doing here?" he says. "You're not supposed to sit and watch TV. Drink up now and go to your room."

I reluctantly finish the rest, get up from the table, and put my cups and dish on the sandwich cart. In the doorway I stop and turn to watch some more TV. He sees me standing there, procrastinating, and says, "No, you can't stay here. Go to bed."

"I'm not tired," I reply.

"Then you'll have to do something else."

"Like what?"

"Read a book or something."

"I can't read. The letters keep moving around."

My medicines make it difficult to see anything up close.

"Nope. Go to bed and rest then."

"But, I told you, I'm not tired."

"Shh!" says someone from the couch.

"You're here to rest. Go to bed now. You're disturbing the other patients with your chatter. They can't hear the TV."

I remain in the doorway, watching.

"Go now. Otherwise I'll have to take you there."

"Sure, you do that," I retort.

Anything to mess with him, like they mess with me. Let them know they're doing a job in this damned place. It's no vacation, is it? The attendant is annoyed that he can't sit in peace and watch Bingo Lotto. Together, we walk down the corridor to my room.

"Are you satisfied now?" he asks me when we arrive.

"Yes. No, I forgot. I need to get a glass of water," I say and turn and walk back to the day room. He sighs and follows me. They've already taken the cart away, with all the glasses and cups, so he goes to the kitchen and fetches me a glass of water.

"Thanks," I say. "That was kind of you. I get a dry mouth from all my meds. Maybe I could have a pitcher in my room?"

"No, let it go, okay?" he says, annoyed.

"Yeah, sure, but you'll just have to come over and fill it a lot. I'll finish this in no time, " I say and empty the glass before his eyes.

He sighs, goes again to the kitchen, and returns with a pitcher full of water.

"So, let's go to your room."

Halfway down the corridor, I say, "I have to pee. Here." I hand him the glass and slip into the bathroom.

I use the restroom. Wash my hands carefully and dry them with paper towels.

"Come on," he says impatiently when I return, since he wants to get back to the TV. He follows me into my room and puts the pitcher on the table.

"There you go."

"Thanks. You guys are so nice here," I say and smile with exaggerated friendliness.

He closes the door and goes back. I watch the clock. It's a few minutes to nine, so I go out again. He hears me and turns around.

"What the hell! Stay in your room!"

"It's nine. I was just going to have a cigarette," I say with a look of innocence.

"Oh, I see," says he, "but then you'll have to go straight back."

"Of course."

Alfred, the sly old man who swears like a trooper, is in the smoking room. I tell him how I'm trying to drive them crazy, and he laughs.

"Yep, you're full of it, aren't you? Lucky there's folks like you around here, so those lazybones have to earn their paychecks."

Many people have disappeared from the ward. I want to leave too. I realize that, if I want to get out of here, it's up to me. It's my responsibility to make it happen, make a change. Even if I don't feel well and would like most of all to go to a rest home/spa, I'll have to pretend. I must obey all the rules, swallow all the pills with a smile, and behave in an exemplary manner. That will be my ticket out of here.

I miss my radio, listening to music. I have a wristwatch that stops if you don't wind it. I tell the night staff it's broken and I need a clock in my room to be able to keep track of smoke breaks and mealtimes. I succeed in convincing the attendant to give me my radio, because it has a clock. It feels like a small victory in spite of the fact that I've given up my struggle. I turn on my radio, turn up the volume, and let myself be sucked into the music, close my eyes and dance around my room. I pretend that all the artists are doing a live broadcast at an arena somewhere in the world. It's a live-aid concert just for me. I feel the applause and the force of it makes me strong.

Ward 22 contains a truly motley group of people. There are patients and caregivers from the four corners of the world. Many of the staff have other professions but are surely working here to earn some extra money. One man, a little younger than me, is an artist. He comes from South America, Bolivia I think. He wonders if he might do my portrait, and I say yes. He's good, sketches quickly in pencil, and captures my soul on paper. A sorrowful woman looks back at me from the drawing.

The artist has one eye that doesn't seem to see. I ask what happened. He tells me that he had an accident as a child and is blind in that eye.

"Can't it be fixed?" I wonder.

He answers that, with today's technology, it's possible.

"Will you do it?'

"No. I've learned to draw with only one eye, and my brain interprets reality from one visual impression. If I get back the sight in my other eye, I'd have to relearn and I'm afraid that I'd lose the ability to draw."

I like his sketch and wonder if he exhibits his pictures somewhere. He says that some of his stuff is on exhibit right now in Central Stockholm, but he's going to take them down tomorrow. I want to go see them. I speak to the staff, and they say they don't think it'll work but they can bring up my request at the doctor's rounds tomorrow.

I wake up at four thirty. The sun is shining, and I'm eager to get out and go to the art exhibit. The first thing I do when I wake up is to ask them when the round will be. They say the doctor will be here around eight. Time passes, and the doctor doesn't come. I'm afraid it will be too late. I pace back and forth and stick my head out my door many times, wondering if the doctor has arrived yet. At last, he comes, and, surprisingly, he says yes. Accompanied by the aide José, I can leave the hospital.

We're late, and we run down to the entrance.

"Come on, let's get a cab," I say, happy as a lark.

"No, it's too expensive," replies José.

"Jeez, I've got money. Come on, let's go. We'll be late."

We hop into a cab outside the hospital's main entrance. What a feeling of liberation, gliding along on a sunny morning like this, through town! There's a lot of activity, and I long to return to reality, to real life outside the hospital walls. When we arrive at the place, we meet the artist, but he has already taken down his works. He tells us that he'll have other exhibits this summer, and he writes down the dates and places for them.

José seems more disappointed than I am. But I explain to him that it's okay. The artist's pictures are still there, and this experience was precious to me. For me, it's fantastic just to get out and move freely among other people. We walk in the sun and buy ice cream before we take the bus back to the hospital.

Now the doctor thinks I've improved and I'm allowed to see my mother. Finally. I've longed for this so much! She comes and picks me up one afternoon. I hug her for a long time. Her soft cheek against mine. It feels so nice to be little again, Mother's little girl.

We drive out to Saltsjöbaden, a very exclusive suburb of Stockholm on the Baltic coast. We park and take a walk. It's a beautiful evening and wonderful to be outdoors. The sun makes the water glitter, and the sea breeze is strong. We sit down at a restaurant and have a light bite, since I've already had dinner. On our way home, I want to stop at a convenience store. I buy cinnamon rolls and cookies for the patients. I want to share a little of my joy at being on the outside.

It's hard to return to the ward. I've had a taste of freedom and I'm still in isolation here. In the evening, when it's time to smoke, I can hardly get out of my room because there's a big black guy parked on a chair outside my door. It scares me, and I wonder who he is.

"Hi, I'm Pendo. I work here."

"I see. Hello, I'm Jenny, and I'm a patient here."

"I know," the dark man answers.

I feel he's a little suspicious, being here. Having him so close feels very invasive. What does he want?

"Why are you sitting outside my door?"

"I work here."

"Yes, you said that. But why are you sitting here? I can hardly get out."

"What are you doing?"

"I'm just going to smoke a cigarette."

He moves aside so I can get out. I walk past him, and he follows me like a shadow. He doesn't accompany me into the smoking room, but I can see him standing outside and watching me through the window. It feels really uncomfortable. When I've finished, I walk to my room and he returns to his chair.

I continue to ask questions, because I wonder why he's here, but he won't answer. Instead, he tells me that he's a construction engineer and works with various development projects in Africa. He goes there from time to time and builds houses, and when he's in Sweden he works here as an attendant.

For the next several days and nights, someone is always seated outside my door. It makes me feel uneasy, and I don't understand it. Later, I find out that, when a patient begins to recover, they increase their vigilance because the patient usually becomes more assertive, which heightens the risk of suicide.

They're letting me spend the night at my mother's house. I've wanted to go there to sleep and have her take care of me for so long. Finally, it's going to happen. In the evening, we go out for dinner with my sisters. It's wonderful to be together again. I haven't been able to speak to them or see them during my isolation.

I tell them about the forced medication and the other awful things I've experienced and cry until my mascara runs in black streaks down my cheeks. Soon we're all sitting there, sobbing in the middle of this hip restaurant in Stockholm called Taste. They can't believe it's true, that that's how the situation was handled. At my mom's, I sleep on the couch in the living room. She pampers me, tucks me in. It's wonderful to be with someone who loves me.

In the morning, her living room is bright with daylight. I wake up at four and can't go back to sleep. I get up and read the paper. When I'm finished, I don't have anything to do and think of walking to the 7-Eleven on the corner to buy fresh bread for breakfast. I get dressed and try to go out but can't open the door. Mother hears me and comes out of her bedroom, drowsy.

"Hi, sweetheart, are you already awake?" she says, bleary-eyed.

"Yes, it got so light out, and I can't go back to sleep once I'm awake."

"Come on, I'll put on some coffee. Are you hungry?"

"Yes, I was going to go to the 7-Eleven to get some bread for breakfast, but the door was locked."

"Yes, you see, I locked the door because the doctor said I have to keep an eye on you. He said you could just disappear."

"Yeah, well, I wasn't going to."

"No, but we have to do as he says. Otherwise, maybe he won't let you visit us again. Now that you've finally been allowed to, we have to abide by their rules. Come on," she says and hugs me, then goes to the kitchen. She puts on some coffee, gets out some bread, and we have breakfast together.

We spend the whole day together. We stroll around and shop a little. Mother will soon be sixty and is planning a party. I look for something to wear and finally find a long red skirt at the H&M downtown. I also buy a pair of white Capris with a colorful flower print. I still feel strange from all the meds. I'm stiff and can't think straight. At lunch, we're going to meet my sisters at a place in Kungsträdgården, the popular central park in Stockholm. We arrive at the huge main square, and suddenly I feel completely panicked. How will I be able to cross that gigantic open space? It's so large and full of people everywhere. My pulse quickens, and I have a hard time breathing. I walk like a robot. It feels as if everyone is staring at me. What'll I do? How will I get through this? Mother feels my anxiety and takes me by the arm. Together, we walk slowly, arms linked, through the park.

That night, I sleep at home in my own house, with my family. It's nice to be home, but it's a mess. Laundry is piled everywhere, and things aren't put away where they should be. I don't feel comfortable in my own home.

Back on the ward, I have a doctor's appointment. I want to reduce my medication. I don't want to have to experience any more panic attacks like the one in Kungsträdgården. At the same time, I know I must keep up my good image and say that I'll gladly follow Dr. K's orders, because I want to be released. He agrees to lower somewhat the dose of Theralen, the neuroleptic that includes a tranquilizer and sleep-inducing agents. Since my short leaves have gone so well, I'll be at home for two nights this coming weekend. I pack and take all my things. Now I'm finished with this place. My committal has been revoked, and in a short while now they won't be able to keep me here against my will.

The weekend goes well. We have dinner one evening at my sister Charlotta's place. My sister Eva and her boyfriend, with whom she's gotten back together, are also there. It's good to see them all, but I feel dulled by the meds and can't keep up with the conversation. Since we were having wine with dinner, I did all I could to avoid taking my evening meds, but Carl kept a check on me and reminded me to take them before we left. I get so sleepy at the table that I sit there nodding. I feel like a damned idiot and have to go lie down on their couch, where I nod off.

On Monday, I'm back at the hospital for observation and blood tests to check on my level of lithium. I get to meet a new doctor, Dr. A, since Dr. K is away. She is petite, with a gracious manner. Her silver hair is styled in a perfect pageboy. Her clothes are tasteful and expensive. Her gaze is sharp, and she seems very intelligent. I tell her that I want to terminate medication, and she agrees to take me off the Nozinan. I want to leave the ward immediately, but she convinces me to stay for a while. She wants to have a talk with Carl before they release me.

From the records:

Psych status: Fully and clearly oriented. A little hyperactive. Rich in association and with insufficient awareness of her illness. Deemed still hyperactive and not really stable.

Together, Carl and I meet with the psychologist on Ward 22 and a counselor to plan the next steps. I absolutely want to be released from the ward but agree to consider going to Sorteria, the open care place, a couple of days a week as they suggest. Tomorrow, we'll pay a visit.

Carl, Angel, and I go to Sorteria together. The place is on the ground floor of an apartment building, not far from where we live. The foyer is full of shoes, with jackets hung on the wall. We hear music. When we enter, I see a guy sitting and playing guitar. Others are sitting, talking, or playing board games. The coffee machine is bubbling in the shared kitchen. So bohemian, I think. There's a sad, loser atmosphere. I immediately feel this is not for me. I have no need to consort with a bunch of depressed people. Sitting and chewing over problems together with them is *not* what I need. We meet a woman counselor. She's nice, explains what they can offer. I'll come three times a week, and I can do what I want. Earlier I'd fantasized about finishing my photo albums here, but I see I can just as well do that at home.

Sometimes they organize outings that I can join. If I want to eat lunch, I'll need to add my name to a list. I'll be assigned a doctor, with whom I'll meet every now and then. We thank her for the visit and go back to the hospital.

The following night, I'm allowed to sleep at home, and then I must go back for observation again before I'm finally released. Now I don't have to sleep in isolation on the ward and can share a room with other female patients. Most of them are new. Since I'll soon be released, I don't get involved and don't speak to them much. I can come and go as I like, and it's a wonderful freedom. I call and book a hair appointment at a salon. I have blond highlights done and wear fresh new spring clothing that my sister Charlotta bought me. I feel like a new person.

Back at the hospital, I have one last doctor's appointment with Dr. A before I'm released. She's just as chic as before. She says the lithium level in my blood is too low to have any effect, and I should increase the dose. It's finally my decision to make, since I'm no longer involuntarily committed, and I say I can't accept that. Dr. A replies that the doctor at Sorteria will probably suggest it too.

"We'll have to see how I feel," I say, though I don't intend to increase my dose. On the contrary, I intend to stop all medication as soon as I'm released, but, of course, I don't say that. She gives me a prescription for several hundred lithium tablets, which I pocket.

Carl picks me up. He's gotten orders from the doctor to drive by the drugstore and pick up the medicine before we go home. There is a familiar foreign pharmacist behind the counter. I've bought antibiotics for my kids from him so many times. This time, I'm ashamed when I give him the prescription. Lithium. God, how awful. I buy all the pills. It's too bad to just throw away so much money, I think, but I keep up the front for Carl's sake.

RELEASED

After five weeks on Ward 22, I've now been released.

After being locked up for more than a month, I have an enormous need to get out, experience the freedom, go to parties, and have fun. On the ward, I had time to think through my life. Since the kids were born, I've been unbelievably tied down, and now I want to change my life and begin again with something new. I can't deal with my sorrow over Lucas's situation; I push it away.

Later, on Friday evening, Carl and I go out for dinner with my sister-in-law, Carin, and her husband. We eat at Bistro Ruby, a nice place in the Old Town. I haven't met or spoken to them in over a month. They wonder a little timidly how it's been. They don't know what to say or how much they can ask without being too indiscreet. I gladly tell them, but how could they ever understand what I've been through? When I get to the part about the forced medication, I can't hold back my tears and I cry again. When I've calmed down, we talk about other things. These are separate worlds, hard to mix.

Carin, who works in our company, tells us about the Clinton event and how successful it was. She had the honor of hosting Bill Clinton at the dinner table. *It could have been me*, I think. I've missed out on a lot. This was the biggest event in Talarforum's history, and it feels bad, like someone stole my thunder.

After dinner, I want to go to Café Opera, a nightclub, and dance. The others aren't in the mood, but I convince them and we walk there in the cool summer evening. There's nothing more beautiful than Stockholm in the summer. The city is buzzing with life, and a festive mood vibrates in the air. There's a line outside of the nightclub, but it doesn't take long before we're inside. We go to the bar and order drinks. I have a frozen margarita, a drink that reminds me of days gone by. I love the taste of salt mixed with lime and tequila, salty and sour.

The music is great, and I want to dance. We take our drinks over to a table near the dance floor and dance together. We really break loose. When the others tire, I dance on alone. The people and music surround me, and I'm intoxicated with life. I could stay out all night, but the others want to go home after a while and we share a taxi. It's very late when we get home. Gunilla, my mother-in-law, is babysitting, and, when we open the door, she rushes up to us.

"Oh, what a relief you're finally home! I was just going to call you. I've been wondering where you were," she says.

"Why?" I ask, slightly irritated by her exaggerated anxiety. "We were out."

"It doesn't matter that you're late. I was just worried that something had happened."

"It must be a pain to always be so worried about everything," I say.

"Yes, it is," Gunilla is ticked off.

"Well, we're so different," I say.

Her solicitousness is suffocating to me now that I've been freed. I need space and want to live life.

The next day, my mother's birthday party is held at my sister's apartment. Mother is sixty years old. I don't have a gift, but I've written a poem for her and framed it. I'm no longer used to being around so many people, and it's a chore to walk around and be nice and pretend how great everything is. Not many people know that I've just been released from a psych ward, but I feel their curious looks about how I'm doing.

Later in the week, I get a letter from Mom. She has sent me a framed photograph of herself with us sisters, meaning well. Everyone looks happy except for me. I look like a hunted animal, caught in an ambush. I hide it in a drawer to avoid looking at it again.

While I was gone, Carl took a leave of absence from work to be at home with the kids. Sara asked about me every day:

"Mommy come home?"

Carl told her I was sick, but that I'd come back when I was well. The minute Lucas heard my name mentioned, he peed his pants. There were no words for him to express his longing. When I got better, Lucas and Sara were allowed to come visit me on a couple of occasions. We often met just outside the hospital, because Carl didn't want them to see me in the hospital environment. After a few visits, Sara asked as they approached the building:

"Mommy lives here?"

They spent their days on outings to beautiful spots in our neighborhood. My mother-in-law was often there, helping with and cuddling the kids. At night, Carl slept with the children in our bed to give them a feeling of security.

BACK TO REALITY

I'm finished taking meds, and I'm back in the real world.

The pills turned me into a medieval knight in a clumsy, rickety, enormous suit of armor. A rusty armor shell that squeaked and complained when I moved. Stiff, steel-backed, and with obvious strain, I was forced to throw one leg in front of the other in order to walk. The armor gave me some protection from the world, but inside it, I was still just as vulnerable. My suit of armor is now gone, and I'm exposed. My soul is exposed, and it's frail and fragile.

My visual impressions are strong, and colors flood my eyes. Sounds are sharp and invade my ears. Maybe it's like being a newborn baby and suddenly meeting the world outside the womb. Food tastes different, explodes in my mouth. My senses are being brutally awakened to life again.

Most of my self-esteem is gone, erased, eradicated. I'm unsure of myself and need to remind myself to be here and now, to exist in reality. I'm at home again, and my children need me, but how will I know what they need? *Look at them, read their faces and see how they are feeling*, I say to myself and make it a habit to stay close and mirror them, to try to capture and fill their needs. The kids force me back to life, and I cannot, will not disappoint them. Their constantly demanding presence causes everything to almost, but just almost, return to normal. Just as if their mother was never away. But I'm no longer the same woman. In spite of the fact that

I've lost some of my self-esteem, I've gained an ability, the will to stand up for what's right for me, make my own decisions, and define boundaries.

Carl asks me if I'm taking my lithium pills, and I lie to his face and say yes, because I know that he and everyone else wants me to continue taking meds. The meds are hidden in the bathroom cabinet, at the top, way back so the kids can't reach them.

I'm still exhausted, but at night I get up anyway when the kids wake up. Carl never wakes, even if the kids are lying beside him in bed, screaming in his ears. I've stopped taking sleeping pills, and when I wake up at night, I'm worried that I won't be able to get back to sleep. I know that I need my sleep. But I do manage to fall back asleep, in spite of my anxiety.

The children cling to me. I understand, because I've been away and they miss their mom, but sometimes I need a little time to myself and then I retreat to the laundry room in the basement. One afternoon, I'm down in the laundry room, ironing. The kids have been with me all day, and it's nice to be alone for a while. I'm standing, ironing and listening to music. I like ironing. It's kind of like meditation. You can ponder and let your thoughts glide. The steam hisses from the iron, and the smell of newly washed clothes pervades the room. When I look out through the little cellar window, I can see how the sun glitters far off on the water in the inlet and how the sailboats' masts sway with the swells. Carl storms in screaming and tears me out of my peaceful mood:

"Is this where you're hiding? Can't you hear that your kids need you?"

"No, what? Are they crying?" I wonder, dejected.

"You probably can't hear anything with this music on. They're screaming like maniacs up there and wondering where their mother is," he says.

"I said I was going down to the laundry room," I say.

"I don't believe you. You just disappear without saying where you're going."

"I do so, but you don't hear it, because you're always sitting inside your man cave watching a movie with the sound turned up."

"That's enough. It's your damned responsibility!" he says. "You can't keep running away all the time." He walks over to the radio on the windowsill, pulls the cord, picks it up, and throws it down onto the tile floor. It smashes on the white tile, and pieces of black plastic fly everywhere. There's silence. We stare at each other, then Carl turns and leaves.

I'm so tired and sad. I can't even find peace and quiet for a few moments. Can't he understand that I need to get away from the kids and be by myself for a while? I cry as I pick up the pieces of the radio and put them in a pile on the counter. How can I stand this? Will we be able to continue living together? I collect myself and go upstairs to the children. They're what's most important. They shouldn't have to suffer because we're fighting. They are already, but I want to protect them from more.

I have a doctor at Sorteria. In early June, I meet Dr. L. She's calm and serious, and her eyes emanate concern. She seems to care about how I'm feeling and asks pertinent questions in order to get an idea of my situation.

From the medical records:

Jenny is markedly unhappy, was in conflict with her husband when she came from her family, and is worried in general about his tendency to anger. Realizes at the same time that her newly developed ability to be clear and manifest her own will, instead of yielding to others, also affects her relationship and can cause conflicts.

I stay in regular touch with Dr. L, but I don't feel the need to do the daily activities at Sorteria. I don't want to associate with a bunch of depressed people and be taken on outings like a child. I want to stand on my own two feet. I need life and joy around me. So, instead, I join a gym in the city. I meet a personal trainer, who goes over the machines and plans a training program for me.

My stamina is not what it used to be, and it's tiring to be with the kids. I try to establish some boundaries and make some demands of Carl to help out more at home. I don't want to return to the way it was before. Carl was almost never with the kids, and he wasn't particularly active doing the household chores. It's summer now and vacation time. He's free. He's here just as much as I am, and we have a shared responsibility.

One morning, I'm in the shower. I hear Sara yelling for me somewhere out there, but I know Carl is there and think he can help her. After a while, the shower door jerks open, and Carl is standing there with Sara in his arms.

"Are you deaf? Don't you hear her yelling?"

"Yes, but you're here," I answer.

"It's not me she wants. Damn, don't you get it?"

"Yeah, but if you don't comfort her at all, she'll never get used to you. You're still her father," I say and close the shower door.

He pulls it open again and tries to hand Sara over to me.

"Here. I can't. You'll have to take her, she needs you."

He always takes the easy way out.

"Do it yourself for once. Try it! I'm standing in the shower, damn it."

"I can't. I tried. You'll have to take her," says Carl and gives me Sara while I'm standing completely wet, with my hair full of shampoo. I take Sara in one arm and follow him, naked, with wet pools of water marking my trail.

"Enough's enough! You can at least do SOMETHING! Here, take Sara now so I can rinse my hair."

He won't take her, so I set her down on the floor next to him and walk back to the shower, while Sara is still crying and calling for me. Carl rushes after me, grabbing my arm and yelling.

"What kind of a fucking mother are you! You're fucking mental! Won't you even take care of your child when she needs you?"

"I do, but I'm in the shower at the moment."

"Dr. K was right. He warned me about you. You're really sick."

The contempt shines through his eyes.

"You are goddamned out of your mind," I say. "I guess it's best if you DO take Sara then," I say, and go back into the shower and slam the sliding door shut.

The tears come. Sick—what's he telling me, really? The door jerks open again. I turn around. Carl is there like a wall, staring at me with disgust. It looks like he wants to spit on me, but he stops himself, slams the door shut, and leaves.

My tears are silent. I close my eyes and turn my face up into the shower spray. I want to rinse off his degradation, but it won't come off. It's too deep to rinse off with a little water. I get out, wrap myself in a towel, and go get Sara, who's still unhappy. I carry her into the bathroom, and we sit on the counter. I sit, rocking her in my embrace, and we hug each other. Her small, soft, chubby arms are around my neck. She's crying so hard that she gets the hiccups. We stay there for a long, long time together on the counter in the bathroom, and after a while she calms down. What shall we do about this? How can we get through it? How am I to get through this?

I almost never get angry, but Carl provokes me and then I get defensive. I'm so unhappy that it's affecting the children. I wish them no harm. I don't want to fight in front of them. If we have things to sort out, then we can do it at night, when the kids have gone to sleep, but sometimes I need to draw the line with Carl and then the children get caught in the middle and that hurts me a lot. Not a day goes by that I don't think that we won't be able to solve this, that we'll have to get a divorce.

One week later, we both visit the doctor at Sorteria. We tell her about our fights. Carl is afraid that I'll leave him and isn't far from thinking of leaving me either. He says how he feels, that he's worried about the kids and that I may have a relapse. He feels powerless, like he's lost control. The kids want most of all to be with me, and when I can't manage, they're very unhappy. Carl can't comfort them. He doesn't want to see them unhappy, and when he can't console them, he wants me to do it. He doesn't want our shortcomings to affect the children, but they do, and it hurts both of us to see it.

From the medical records:

In spite of the charged atmosphere, Jenny has a calmer demeanor today, more collected than when she was released. She expresses sorrow and disappointment, as well as anger, but the basic atmosphere seems neutral. Nothing psychotic evident.

Previously, Carl gave me my sense of security, but now I have no security anywhere.

I don't have many close friends I can talk to, and at the same time, I don't want to badmouth Carl with the friends I have, nor with my family. It's my relationship with Carl we're talking about and not their relationships with him. I'm afraid they'll hurt more than help. They would want to protect me from Carl, take me away from there, and make the rift between us even greater. Somewhere inside me, I think, I hope that we'll still be able to make it through this. Deep down, we have a great, mutual love, but it's overshadowed by our problems and worries about Lucas. Divorce is not a good choice. The children would suffer too much. The thought of leaving, breaking away, and fleeing to a new life is tempting, but it's too simple.

We're under pressure in our current situation, but we also discuss things like two reasonable people and decide to go to couples therapy. We visit a psychologist at the children's autism center. She sees parents who've recently received a diagnosis that their children have functional disorders. The woman who greets us is in her fifties. She's dressed in beige linen, is calm, has a pleasant manner, and exudes thoughtfulness. She asks us to tell her about our situation, and we both instinctively feel a lot of trust in her. We share our problems, and she bounces them back and gets us to see them from another perspective, so we can find ways to handle different situations. Carl realizes that his anxiety is turning into anger toward me, and we get a little closer. We have a loving foundation, but it's hidden far away and it'll take time to find it again.

We meet with her a few times, but then one day she cancels because she has a back problem. We're offered a replacement, but we decline, since we want to continue with the same psychologist. When her back problem drags on, she goes on extended sick leave and we don't see her again, but she gave us tools to deal with our conflicts and we don't feel the need to see anyone else. We find our own solutions and slowly begin to regain trust in our relationship.

I've been placed on sick leave for the summer and received a doctor's certificate that I'm supposed to send in to the national health insurance bureau. On the certificate, written by Dr. K, it gives the reason as psychosis. Am I still sick now, as Carl said? I need to know more and ask to see Dr. L at Sorteria and read my medical records. She hands me the records and lets me have peace and quiet to go through them. There are fourteen typed pages. On the first page, from the visit to the ER at Saint Göran Hospital, I read:

Assessment:

Previously essentially healthy patient with suspected psychosis-like experience. Fluctuating and emotionally unstable condition, confused. Assessed to fill the criteria for involuntary commitment according to paragraph 4, commitment.

A few pages later, Dr. K writes that I have a reactive psychosis, caused by a life crisis in combination with exhaustion. As I continue, the words stir many strong emotions. I remember the unspeakable terror I felt before the forced medication and the degradation I was subjected to, which make me question the mental health care system.

When I've finished, I ask Dr. L, "Am I sick now?"

"No, you're not. What we see is that you had a reactive psychosis that was caused by a great crisis regarding your son's condition, combined with lack of sleep and total exhaustion. You hit a wall, and there was no way to go on. Your body was forced to react in some way to stop you. There is no indication you'll become ill again. However, it's important now that you take care of yourself, that you eat well and get lots of sleep. Lack of sleep for a long period is dangerous for anybody. You held out for a really long time with very little sleep, and it had its consequences."

Her answer calms me, and I ask her to write down all the medicines I was given during my time in the hospital. It's a long list:

Nozinan
Theralen
Inderal
Tegretol
Disipar
Nitrazepam
Stesolid
Zyprexa
Imovane
Cisordinol-Acutard
Lithionit

At home, I look them up online in FASS, the Swedish pharmaceuticals directory. As I read, I get chills recognizing one side effect after another. It says that akathisia, which I got from the injection, can lead to suicidal behavior and I understand why. It was really that bad.

I read about psychoses on the Internet. The reactive psychosis consists of serious "benign" psychoses, triggered by a high-pressure situation, sometimes combined with physical exhaustion or illness. They are much more common than other, more serious kinds of psychoses. I order books about various mental states and psychoses. When the books arrive and I read them, I realize that I've been through a temporary psychosis triggered by a life crisis, and that I'm neither sick nor autistic, nor do I fit any other diagnosis. I wanted so badly to find answers to my son's problem, and when there were none, I put the blame on myself. Now I understand that I was wrong, that it's not my fault, and my self-reliance slowly begins to return.

During the summer, we take a vacation to Minorca, a wonderful island next to Mallorca in the Mediterranean Sea. Minorca is smaller, more peaceful, and perfect for families with kids. There are many tiny inlets with lovely, untouched beaches to discover. We stay in an apartment on the second floor. We asked for a balcony, wiser for experience from our previous vacations when we stayed on the ground floor. We had a terrace then, and it was impossible to leave the door open to let air in. Lucas would be gone in the blink of an eye. He was fearless and always ran off without checking if we were following him. He loved water and would immediately make his way toward the pool. He was only two, so he couldn't swim. Keeping watch on him was a constant chore. Now he's three and a half and still can't swim, but he can't get down from the balcony.

It's been a good day, without any giant mishaps or incidents. The days have gone well, but the nights are another matter. We dread each evening. Sometimes it's calm, but sometimes it gets chaotic. Lucas wakes up often several times every night, but not quite as often as before. Now that he's a little older, he can sleep at least an hour and a half at a time. When he wakes up, though, he gives a shout and then we need to be fast, get to him, and hold him so he feels that someone is there with him. Tonight he goes to sleep without a problem at around eight o'clock. He was exhausted. He has been in the water more than on land all day. He doesn't seem to feel the chill like we do.

Tonight we're not fast enough when he wakes up. He doesn't go back to sleep. He becomes hysterical. Nothing can comfort him. It's as if he can't receive our tenderness and closeness. He's so completely impossible to reach. We do everything possible. We stroke him, carry him, we sing songs, we give him something to drink, we put him back to bed, remove the blankets because maybe he's hot, and this goes on hour after hour.

I read once in a book about children that, almost immediately after birth, the parents learn to recognize their child's cries and the reasons for them. The child has different cries for hunger, wanting to be held, being too hot, and so on. When Lucas was smaller, I was always baffled and couldn't understand why it was impossible to discern what he wanted. Now I know better. We can't interpret his signals. He isn't like other children. Even as an infant, he showed limitations in his ability to communicate.

Tonight is one of those evenings when the crying just goes on. Carl carries him until he can't manage any longer, and then I continue. We take turns trying to get him to calm down. Suddenly there's a knock on the door. I look over at Carl. We don't want to open it. Another knock on the door. Go away, I think. Can't you hear we're busy?

Carl says, "Open it. You're better at handling people. I get so angry."

I open up. A dark-haired woman my age is standing there. Her skin is light-colored and freckled from the sun.

"Can you please try and keep your child quiet? He is keeping our children awake. They can't sleep with all the noise."

She looks irritated and tries to look in over my shoulder. Carl and Lucas have gone into our bedroom, so they're not in view, but you can still hear them.

"We're doing our best," I answer.

"Well, try bloody harder. We're on vacation, you know."

I close the door and feel tears running down my cheeks.

LUCAS STARTS PRESCHOOL

It's approaching the end of summer, and autumn comes quietly. My hospital stay was a time-out, and, for a little while, I could forget my son and his handicap. However, reality soon catches up with us, and now it's time for us to deal with Lucas's continued training and introduction to preschool. Carl is back at work. I'll stay home for the autumn, to rest, take it easy, and recover while the kids are in their respective preschools. Carl has promised to work a little less in order to be at home more with the kids and me. We want to rebuild our family.

We have an appointment for an assessment at the autism center. We meet a speech therapist, a kind but stern woman with gray hair, approaching the age of sixty. She's going to observe Lucas while he plays. Lucas follows her into a room, and Carl and I accompany a psychologist and a counselor into an adjacent room, which has windows looking into the room where Lucas is. He can't see us, because the window is one-way and his side has a mirror on it. The speech therapist tries to get Lucas involved in various activities. Suddenly, he calls out, "Mommy?" and gives the therapist a questioning look.

She assures him that I'll be coming soon and he's satisfied with that answer, but she has her hands full keeping him focused on the activities she has chosen for him.

A couple of weeks later, we're back without Lucas. The speech therapist tells us what she's seen during her observation of him, based on which she's planned an intervention. We'll work with the basics of communication. This includes everything from exercises for mouth motor function, like blowing Styrofoam balls back and forth to each other, to practicing taking turns in the form of simple games.

In August, Lucas begins acclimatization at the preschool. It's a Montessori preschool and I'm worried about what will happen. Montessori methods are based on the child's own initiative in taking an interest in things, which is a nice thought, but Lucas isn't like everybody else. It's hard for him to get involved of his own volition and he needs help getting started and sticking with an activity, which is completely contrary to the school's pedagogy. We chose it because Lucas's cousins go there. Besides, it's a small school, and the staff seems to be very invested and have a great rapport with the kids. They treat every individual with respect.

Lucas receives a full-time aid, Lina, a woman my age, who has two children of her own. Her youngest daughter is like my Sara. She's worked at the preschool for a time and knows how they work there. She's pleasant and friendly and approaches Lucas the right way. He immediately likes her, but she has her work cut out for her.

In the preschool, there is a playroom and a classroom. In the classroom, all the Montessori materials and playthings are available. Lucas loves beads and other small, glittery objects, and he rushes around like a playful puppy, making messes and spilling things onto the floor in his quest for treasures. In the playroom he throws Legos around, and in the pillow room he destroys the forts the other kids are building. At circle time, he refuses to participate, and at the lunch table it's even worse. I'm beginning to wonder if we've made the right choice. Will it really work out? Maybe Lucas should go to a special preschool instead? But we've fought so hard to get him into this one.

A special needs teacher from the autism center comes for a day. She observes and later makes suggestions to adapt the activities so that they will suit Lucas. The speech therapist from the center meets Lina and gives her exercises she can do with Lucas.

Acclimatization takes three weeks. For Lucas, who's now close to four years old, it's a big step to be away from me, participate in a group of children, and be taken care of by adults he doesn't know and who don't understand him. Because he doesn't know many words, he often gets angry, yells, and spits on others out of pure frustration. When Sara and I come to pick him up in the afternoons, he's standing at the gate, waiting for us. I can see him from far off, his blond hair sticking up over the edge of the fence, and it's heartrending. I see and hear how the other children are playing and running around the yard, but my Lucas is standing there all alone, waiting and waiting to get out of there, to go home.

His face lights up when he sees us, and we walk home together. Sara sits in the stroller, and Lucas walks. We usually walk both to and from the preschool. It's not far, and only takes ten minutes when I walk by myself. When we walk together it can take an hour, because Lucas walks so slowly.

Sometimes I see the patients from Ward 22 when we're out walking. I may meet Fredrik, the schizophrenic, on the way to preschool with his son in a stroller. We exchange greetings and smile in silent understanding. We share a secret privy to no one else in the neighborhood, except for our loved ones. I often see Alice, the tough lady in a tie from Ward 22 who looks more like a man. The first time, she did a double take when she saw me, but she didn't say a thing and I think she had trouble placing me. Sometimes she looks pretty healthy, but other times she shuffles along with a walker. I also bump into some of the staff. Some must live in our area. It feels strange to see them on the outside. They often act embarrassed and don't know how to behave.

Lucas and I walk everywhere. He isn't as physically active as other kids. He doesn't run around and play like they do, and for me it's important that he get exercise. I notice that he's calmer then. He often protests in the morning, but I persist, and finally it becomes a routine and our walks become a pleasant activity. We discover things, pick berries, gather leaves and rocks, and jump in puddles, and Lucas becomes a good walker. When the preschool goes on outings, he's the one who walks the farthest without complaining.

Lucas says no to most things. I know him and know that you sometimes have to force him to try new things. Otherwise, he'll never learn them. His resistance level is high, but when he gets over the threshold, it's usually okay and he finds new interests. Lina, his aide, is a little too lax with him. She's been schooled in the Montessori method and believes that the will and drive to learn must come from Lucas. We've received exercises from the speech therapist that she's supposed to do with Lucas, but many times he's refused and she respects his will and then there's no training going on.

Lucas's development is slow, and we hire a special needs teacher to work with him after preschool. She comes once a week, and they work up in the loft, a small apartment we've built over the garage. Fredrik, Lucas's previous "coach," has begun working as a schoolteacher, but he also comes over now and then and helps out on the weekends.

In late autumn, Lucas begins to wet his pants again. He's been dry since last summer, but now he wets himself every day. I'm worried that he doesn't like preschool. I meet with Lina to discuss it. She tells me that it's the same thing every day. Things go well when they're inside during the morning. After lunch, all the kids go to the lavatory and then out in the yard to play. Lucas goes to the lavatory too, but as soon as they are outside, he wets his pants. He's allowed to go inside and take off his rain breeches and change pants. She feels it would be good if I bought an extra pair of rain breeches, so there is always a dry pair on hand. When she says it, I understand what the problem may be and say, "Lina, can't you try letting Lucas go out tomorrow without the rain gear?"

"No, I can't. All the children must wear rain gear. That's the way it is in this school."

"I know that. But we need to find out why Lucas is wetting his pants. I think it has something to do with the rain gear. It may be a way for him to avoid having to use them, and that's why he's peeing in them."

"Do you think so?"

"Yes, maybe. I know that he doesn't like wearing rain gear."

"It's usually a struggle to get them on. Okay, we'll try tomorrow and see what happens."

Next day, Lucas is allowed to go out without his rain gear and he doesn't wet his pants, nor does he the next day or the next. Lucas doesn't use many words and has a hard time communicating, so he uses the tricks he knows to get others to react. What we must do is try to interpret this.

During the autumn, Lina is often ill. The preschool has an on-call system, using parents to cover for staff who are sick. All the parents have signed up for different days and, to begin with, they call in the parent who is on the list to help with the children and someone from the staff takes care of Lucas. This works most times, but sometimes, as when they're heading out into the woods for a hike, they call me and ask if I won't come pick Lucas up. He doesn't like the woods, and the preschool doesn't feel they have the expertise to deal with him when he protests.

Finally, I have to sub for Lina every time she's gone, because the other parents can't take leave from work. They'll lose income. I've begun a course called Child Language Development at the university and won't lose any income by being at the preschool, but still I'm sacrificing my time.

In December, Lina's daughter gets sick, and she's gone the whole month. This continues on and off during the spring semester—I'm Lucas's teacher during the daytime and in the evenings at home, I'm his mother. Some days, I can't manage being "teacher," so Lucas stays home with me instead and we do his exercises up in the loft above the garage.

The preschool blames the lack of funding for this and doesn't want to bring in a substitute for Lina. I feel powerless. I know that the school regards Lucas as demanding, and, even though they don't say it out loud, I understand that they don't think Lucas fits well into their activities and would prefer that he leave the school. He disturbs their way of doing things, and they've had no experience dealing with a special needs child, so they have no tools for it. I cry silently to myself because I want him to fit in, to be like everyone else. I don't want him to go to a special needs daycare and, besides that, his cousins are here and he likes them a lot. He's been granted a one-on-one paraprofessional by the municipal office, and when Lina is there, he's fine, but now she's away more than she's present and he needs someone at his side. One afternoon, when I arrive to the preschool to pick up Lucas, a girl comes running and shouts to me before I've even gotten through the gate.

"Do you know what happened today?"

"No . . .what happened today?" I say happily, while I open the gate and enter the yard.

"Lucas cut Anna's finger and she got a big sore. She cried for a really long time."

"Oh, my," I say and look at her. "He probably didn't mean it."

"And do you know what *else* he did?" says a boy who has come running up to us.

"No," I answer and would rather not know or have to listen at all.

"He bit Gustav's arm, and it almost bled. Gustav's got bite marks on his arm from Lucas's teeth. I could count eight of them."

"That's not allowed," I say, because I can't think of anything better. I continue into the yard with my head held down.

While I'm walking along the gravel path up to the entrance, several children approach and they all want to tell me what Lucas did today. Each word from these upset children hits me like a fist, right in the gut. I hurriedly approach the door. I want only to retrieve Lucas and take him away, take him home to our secure world. When I step inside, I'm met by Vera, a fantastic preschool teacher who's always full of energy. I ask timidly what happened, since Lucas cut someone with a pair of scissors and bit another child.

She calms me and says, "Oh, it's not that bad. It happens sometimes. Lucas can get a little angry when he doesn't understand or if someone does something to him that he doesn't like. But that happens to all kids."

It's good to hear that she sees Lucas as one of the others and doesn't treat him as a special case. I feel better. Maybe it's not that serious.

"Was Lina here today?" I ask.

"No. Her daughter is sick again."

That evening, the preschool principal calls home.

"Something serious has happened, and we need to talk," she says as soon as I answer. She recounts in detail how Lucas behaved and how he injured the other children. She says the other children are beginning to be afraid of Lucas and avoid him when he approaches them.

"We can't continue like this," she says. "Soon he may harm someone seriously."

"No," I say, agreeing with her. "But that's why Lucas has an aide to help him and support him in difficult situations."

"Yes, but her child is very ill now, and we can't guarantee that there will always be someone at Lucas's side. That's not the way it works with us."

Between the lines, I hear her saying that we should look around for another preschool for Lucas.

I'm struggling with everything and everyone. I'm hugging my son with one arm and holding a sword in the other, fighting my way forward. We're met with blows from all directions, and I defend us as well as I can. I try to keep Lucas out of it, but we both get hurt and, when he's hurt, it affects me doubly.

I call my mother-in-law and am swallowing my tears, I tell her what's happening, that they're trying to push us out. Gunilla has worked in preschools for many years, and before she retired she was the superintendent of preschools in the municipal administration. She advises us to ask for a meeting with the head of preschools and the municipal preschool representative. We do this the same week, and at the meeting we explain the situation and how sorry we are that the preschool hasn't been able to make it work. We total the number of times that Lucas's aide has been absent. When the woman from the municipal office learns the actual situation, she reacts vigorously and tells the preschool principal that they can be reported for this. When we're finished, the municipal rep asks the preschool principal to stay behind. I don't know what's said, but afterwards Lucas receives a new aide, Penny. Penny is nice, and Lucas is quickly drawn to her. He is more secure and the accidents stop. She works with him on his exercises. He learns them quickly and needs new ones, but appointments with the speech therapist are tough to schedule. Lucas's progress is slow, and his speech is not developing.

LETTER TO LUCAS

Lucas,

It's increasingly obvious that you're different. You're over four years old, and you say almost nothing. When someone speaks to you, you turn away or look straight through him or her, as if the words become letters that fall apart in the air and fly past you. Voices are white noise that you block out and don't take note of.

Some people seem a little embarrassed or offended when you don't react, as if they're ashamed. Others joke about it and say, "Me? I'm an old fart, not much to pay attention to."

Lucas, what do you hear? What registers with you? What do you take in? You are a riddle. A beautiful riddle. You hold your well-formed head at an angle sometimes, as if you were listening to something no one else hears. Sometimes, your serious gaze rests far away and sees what no one else sees. Where are you in those intervals? You disappear to another world, far away, one that only you have the key to. Your own world. I hope it's a good world, but I also want to share our world with you. I tug and pull at you to get you to join, to establish contact, but sometimes you're like mercury that just runs off, glides away, and then it's impossible to reach you.

If I want to reach you for sure, I can say, "Let's play chase!"

You brighten up, the spark in your eyes lights up and you're immediately with me. However, it's always on your terms, never on mine.

Sometimes you disappear in another way. You "stim," as it's called. You stimulate your senses in various ways. It could be by spinning around on the floor until you're completely dizzy, or jumping on couches or beds. Your own bed has collapsed. At preschool, we've brought you a small trampoline you can jump on whenever you need to release some energy. At home, we have a large trampoline in the yard, where you can bounce way up to the sky and almost grab the branches in the nearby tree.

You play with your field of vision and stimulate your visual impressions by holding up your fingers in a certain pattern in front of your eyes or by looking through pieces of glass that you find on the ground. Other times, you choose to close down, like when noises become too loud or too sharp. Then you cover your ears and close it out. If someone coughs or sneezes, you can start to cry.

You seem to have a very good memory. You know all of your video films by heart. You run and hide before the scary part comes, and you laugh beforehand at the things you think are funny. You choose the correct film just by looking at the cassette covers, and you seem to have memorized what the word looks like, because you can't read. You remember the roads we drive and can get upset if we turn in the wrong direction. Is it because you're used to taking one route, or is it because you want to go somewhere in particular? I ask you, but I never get an answer.

You often encounter the world with a no, and we struggle together on an uphill slope. You scream your way to the top, while I take turns pulling and pushing. Finally, we reach the top, and sometimes we're lucky enough to find a downhill slope that we both enjoy running down. Other times, it's just a straight stretch, or a hilltop and then another uphill climb. But I'm learning that there are no shortcuts if you are to exist in our world. We must go forward together. I do all I can to make your journey easier, I hope so anyway, even if my gnawing conscience is there, like a yoke I always carry. One can always do more and better, and I certainly want nothing else when it comes to you and your future, but there must also be some balance. I must be able to manage going on living.

I try to help you through your everyday life as well as I can, to listen to what you want and mean. We use many pictures when we talk to each other. When we're going out, I show you pictures so you'll know what you can expect. I bring the camera and take pictures of new places, new things we do, so we'll be able to look at the pictures and share an experience again and have something to talk about. You have your own pictures to show if you want to have or do something, but you also use the few words you know. I know you so well that one single word from you can become a long sentence for me, while others are in complete darkness, trying to understand your attempts to communicate.

How will you get by in this world?

I take you on activities so you'll get to do the same things as other kids. We go to the kids' pool, and you love that. Water is your second element. You glide around like a sea lion, splashing, snorting, and laughing.

Once, we try an outing adapted for children with autism, arranged by the National Autism Society. We go to the Natural History Museum to see an Imax movie. We park and walk up the hill to the museum. Carl and I snatch glances at other autistic children, both young children and teenagers. This is a new world for us. What can we expect farther down the road in life? We both do and don't want to know. Walking up to the museum, we sneak looks at the others. There's a boy in front of us, and you can see right away from his movements that he's autistic. I would never have noticed it before, but now it's like we've become experts. We see them everywhere— these kids and adults with autism. It took us several years to discover that you had it, but then we didn't know what we know today.

I notice that Carl is feeling a little uncomfortable. He's not at home in this situation. I'm more curious but also sad. How is it going to be? How will you develop? At the movie, I see a boy who just sits rocking back and forth and sometimes making some noises.

The handicap is so obviously tragic when you're on a mass outing like this. I don't want you to belong to a special group. I don't want to see you in any other way than I see Sara. I don't want your autism to become your identity.

We don't participate in any more activities like that, but it's a strain to be with you among others who don't know you, because you're different and they can't understand. You probably don't notice it, but we do. Carl avoids it, finds it difficult. He's an innately shy person, and it gets more acute when he has to do something with you. Maybe in front of other people he thinks it's hard that you're different. It's sad that it has to be that way. I don't care what others think, but it is a strain always having to deal with how your surroundings react.

You look like everyone else. Your handicap isn't visible. This is both a blessing and a curse. A blessing because it means that you don't always get stared at, and a curse because you encounter less understanding when something happens that you can't deal with. When you have a meltdown in a shop, I can feel the dirty looks come our way. Looks that mean to convey that I haven't brought you up well, my child, that I should handle you better, admonish you, talk you into better behavior. But many times, it's impossible to know why you're screaming and impossible to deal with it. In the United States, they have what's called autism awareness cards. They're small cards, sort of like business cards, with an explanatory text. From the card, one can read that the child has autism, a handicap that makes it difficult to deal with various situations. He isn't spoiled or rowdy, and we're not bad parents because we don't tell him to behave. He's doing his best, so be patient. If you want to know more about autism, go to this website. The cards are supposed to be distributed when there's a situation and you feel people are staring or questioning your actions. But I don't want to have cards to give away. It would feel wrong. I don't want to treat you in any way different from Sara. I don't want you to have to feel accused, feel different. To me, you're not different. To me you're just you. You're my son, Lucas, whom I love.

You don't understand when I explain things, and then misunderstandings happen that are hard to undo. You can also be frightened by different things or react to noises or smells. There was one period when you refused to walk by the produce section in a certain store, which made it hard to shop. As soon as we approached that corner, you went stiff and didn't want to go any closer. If I tried, you screamed and ran in a different direction. I don't know if it was the smells, the colors, or something else that scared you.

Another time, I was going to work out with my sister at a gym. We brought you kids along so you could all play with each other in the playroom. I didn't think you'd play with the others, but there was a ball pit that I thought you might like, and then they showed cartoons and you like that. Not live-action movies with real actors; it has to be animated movies. The gym is located in a basement, and on the walls of the stairwell they've painted different children's book characters, like Pippi Longstocking, Alfie Atkins, Winnie the Pooh and his friends, and many others. When you saw all the familiar characters from your movies, you went stiff with fear and screamed. You refused to go down there. You covered your eyes while I carried you down. We went back there a second time, but the same thing happened again. The third time, I showed you the picture from the playroom with the ball pit and you started to scream because you remembered those characters so well. Then I gave up.

Sometimes, we go to an activity center, Nicki's Adventure Park. There's a jumping castle, a gigantic, inflated slide, and play equipment with ball pits, slides and obstacles. It's a place you love, and it suits you perfectly. Here, you can play and be with other kids in an environment you know and like. You run around for hours, and sometimes, all sweaty, you seek us out to have a drink of juice and cool down. You play by yourself but gladly will wrestle with me on the soft mattresses or build high towers out of the big, colorful pillows. If I'm not close by, you find one of the other adults and begin to climb on them because you want to wrestle. I quickly come over and explain to you that you can wrestle with Carl and me but not with others whom you don't know, but I'm not sure you understand what I mean. You don't have social boundaries and at any time can walk up to people you don't know. People feel you're a little too pushy and intrusive, and we try to get you to understand that you need to treat people differently, that you can't simply approach people you don't know in new places.

At Nicki's, all the kids must wear socks. You hate socks and refuse to wear them, and we let you run around without them. One time, one of the staff comes up and tells you that you must wear socks, and you laugh and want to wrestle. I can see that you don't understand. I walk up to her and say that you're allergic and can't wear tight-fitting socks. Small white lies are often useful to make your day easier.

You are fascinated by smoke. When we're in a parking lot, I have to hold onto your hand so you don't run up to cars, squat down by the exhaust pipe, and observe the smoke that comes out. You think it's great when Carl smokes a cigar. You want him to blow smoke in your face. Once, outside a shop, a man sat on a park bench, smoking. You rushed up to him and pulled his arm and wanted him to blow smoke at you. The guy was really freaked out by it and looked uncertain how to react. I was afraid he'd hit you or do something, because he looked so frightened. You got too close, did something unexpected and made him insecure.

You mean no harm, but sometimes things go wrong. It must be hard for you to get a grip on the world and how it works. I want to help you along the way and will do my best to make it easier for you. You are my son, and I love you just the way you are.

MEDICAL EXAMINATION

Lucas has to have a medical examination at the hospital. We had the psychological part done privately, but whether or not he has any medical problems remains to be determined. They take blood for tests, and Lucas gives a urine sample. We have to wait for the results, but after a few weeks we receive a letter saying that the urine test for metabolic disorders is normal. The blood test shows that Lucas isn't gluten intolerant and his thyroid levels are normal. They've done a DNA analysis, and he has a normal male chromosome makeup, not fragile X syndrome, which is a chromosome disease that causes autistic spectrum disorders.

Lucas has to return once and to have an EEG done. More than twenty small metal electrodes are fastened to special spots to his scalp. The electrodes are connected to a machine that draws a computer picture of his electrical brain activity. I'm anxious about how it will go, whether he'll cooperate or not, but they have a TV and he sits watching a movie while they do the examination. He finishes it without much protest. The EEG shows no brain injuries and no signs of epilepsy, which is common in autism.

While there, we're offered the chance to do a CT scan of Lucas's brain, but we're hesitant and say no. A CT scan is an X-ray, and many small rays would be sent to the brain from different angles. Lucas would need to be sedated in order to lie still, and we're fearful about how the sedation and the radiation, which is quite a bit higher than in ordinary X-rays, would affect him. For weeks afterwards, I discuss this with Carl back and forth, and finally we come to the conclusion that we should have the examination done. None of the other tests have revealed anything, and we feel it's our duty to Lucas and ourselves to do the tests that are offered in order to find out whether there is some explanation for his handicap. He could have a brain tumor, and you need to X-ray to find that out. It's unlikely. The doctors say that there are no signs pointing to a tumor, but we still want to be on the safe side.

In the morning, I show Lucas a picture of the doctor and the hospital and tell him that we'll be going there to do a test. Lucas can't eat any breakfast, since he's going to be sedated. I bring out a Band-Aid soaked with local anesthesia and show him how it sticks to the backsides of his hands. He doesn't like to wear Band-Aids and fights it, but finally he agrees to let me put a little anesthetic cream on the back of his hands and then put the special Band-Aid on top. They need to sit for an hour to numb the places where the nurse will be putting in a port for the sedative.

They find no brain tumors, and nothing else aberrant when they scan his brain. After the medical investigation, we still have no answers. It feels like we've gone full circle, returning to the place where we began. We continue to turn all the possible causes inside out. Is he autistic because of a bump on the head when he was tiny? When he was only a few months old, I brought him with me on the bus. For part of the way home, I planned to change to a train, so I gathered my things and prepared to get off. The bus stopped suddenly, the brakes squealed, and people went flying from their seats and fell all over the place. I threw myself after the baby carriage but not in time, and it fell over. Lucas, who was sleeping inside, fell out and landed on his head. He woke up and began to scream. I picked him up and tried to comfort him. Other passengers helped me with the carriage and wondered if they could help in any way. Crying, I called Carl and wondered what to do.

"Call the hospital," he said, and I did. I spoke to the ER staff and told them what had happened. They didn't think I needed to come in and said that children are resilient and usually make it through falls okay, but I should be attentive and make sure he didn't become sluggish or begin vomiting. Lucas calmed down after a little while, and I sat on a bench to nurse him. I took the train home. Lucas seemed fine, and we never visited the doctor. I now replay his fall repeatedly in my mind. It was in the winter, and he was wearing thick overalls complete with a hood, and he lay in a padded bag that fell with him. I hope it cushioned his fall somewhat.

I search everywhere for explanations. I read in the newspaper that smoking can cause autism. Maybe I smoked at parties once or twice before I knew I was pregnant. What if I caused my child's handicap?

The causes of Lucas's autism could be any number of things, and we speculate about them, wanting to find solutions, yet realizing that knowing the answer may not do any good or change anything for Lucas. There are no known cures for autism at this time, so what does it matter if you know the cause? Common sense tells us one thing, but emotions say another and we want answers.

There are numerous theories as to why children are autistic. Something might have happened during pregnancy or birth. Ours was a long delivery. Lucas was completely blue when he was born, and they sprayed oxygen over him so he would wake up. Carl is convinced that he had a lack of oxygen to his brain, and he thinks that's the explanation. I'm not so sure and continue to ponder. I read a lot about different theories of how autism appears. I have a library full of books, and the Internet is an infinite source of information.

At the Swedish Board of Health and Welfare website, I find a syndrome under the heading of Lesser Known Handicaps, called Catch-22, that I think Lucas might have. The syndrome is caused by a loss of a small piece of the chromosomes in chromosome pair 22. The symptoms and their gravity can vary. A person with mild symptoms may not even know that he or she has Catch-22, while in others it is a lot more noticeable. The symptoms that fit Lucas are heart disease, problems with infections, speech difficulties, learning difficulties, and aberrant behavior. At Lucas's four-month physical examination, his doctor discovered a heart murmur. We were sent to a cardiologist at the Astrid Lindgren Children's Hospital, who examined his heart with ultrasound. They discovered that Lucas has a constricted aorta. It did not need surgery, but he still goes in for regular checkups to make sure it's not getting worse.

I call Lucas's doctor, Dr. F, who is in charge of the medical investigation, and wonder if she's tested Lucas for Catch-22.

"No," she answers. "I haven't. We've done a chromosome analysis, but you can't usually see Catch-22 there."

"I've read some about it and think that much of it fits Lucas. Catch-22 can look like autism," I say.

"Yes, except I didn't think he showed the symptoms that characterize the syndrome."

I immediately begin to list the symptoms that fit.

"He has a constricted aorta, he's been prone to infections. I don't know how many ear infections he's had. He's had false croup on several occasions, and we've had to go the hospital. He has difficulty speaking, and he has some odd behavior. He doesn't sleep well. I see a lot of things that correspond."

"Yes, there's a lot there," she concedes, "but these children usually also have a characteristic appearance."

"That's true," I respond, "but it doesn't necessarily have to be that way. Some people have the syndrome without even knowing it. Besides, Lucas has slightly special ears," I say, because I know all the symptoms by heart. They look like cauliflower ears.

"We can do a blood analysis to see if he has Catch-22," she says. "I don't think he does, but if you're unsure and are worried about it, I think we should do it."

"Yes, that would be good. Otherwise, I'll always wonder."

We make an appointment, and Lucas lets them take some blood. When the doctor sees Lucas, she says, "Yep, you were right about his ears. They're a little different."

Lucas's ears are large, soft, and rounded. His outer ears look like small bowls.

I wait for the test results, almost hoping that he has Catch-22, so I can put it behind me and not have to wonder. After a few weeks, we receive a letter that says that Lucas's blood tests were normal and he does not have Catch-22. We're forced to continue living in the dark. It doesn't matter to Lucas what the cause might be. Not now, while he's little. With time, as he matures and understands more, he may want to have answers, but the most important thing for him now is to have our love and to feel loved as he is. However, both Carl and I know that love is not enough. Much, much more than that is needed for Lucas to have a good life, and I hope we can manage it.

ONE MORE CHILD

Life rolls on, and slowly Carl and I become closer again. We talk a lot about what happened and begin to understand each other's actions. Emotions, such as fear and inadequacy, often got in the way of common sense and we projected our own weaknesses onto each other by attacking, but time has given us perspective. It's easier to look back and see what happened with more clarity than we had amid the chaos. The wounds we inflicted on each other were deep and will take time to heal, but slowly we rekindle the love that we once had for each other. Sometimes, we talk about the time when I was in the hospital, and I feel Carl should have done more to get me out of there. He explains that he couldn't because I'd been committed and wasn't allowed to be moved. Eva had found a place for me I was released, but by then we didn't need it. I got well faster than we expected. The injection I was forced to take also left its mark, and every time we talk about it, I cry. But the crying is a way to work through the experience and put it behind me, in order to be able to move forward.

For Easter vacation, we go to Tenerife in the Canary Islands. We travel with my in-laws and their kids and rent a large house up in the mountains above Las Americas.

Sara loves to be with her cousins. Jesper is a couple of years older, and Anna is four years older. It's the closest Sara can get to having normal siblings. Lucas is her brother and a large part of her life, but they don't play together like she does with Jesper and Anna. Sara is still small, not yet three, but how she loves to play! She's an early speaker, which gives her an advantage, and her need for play, interaction, and acknowledgment is transformed into an enormous energy, a never-ending force. She absorbs, clings, and never wants to stop, because she's getting a response. She is being acknowledged, and our little daughter is growing. It's not easy for her to have a brother like Lucas. He loves her, but he's the way he is, special. It's hard to relate to someone and only give, give, give while receiving only a fraction in return and sometimes being totally rejected.

I admire Sara when, time after time, she tries to interact with Lucas, but her needs are very different than his. Playing comes naturally to her as an unquestioned part of life, necessary in order to grow. But for Lucas, it doesn't exist, and she receives blows or screams and is sometimes completely ignored. She's stubborn, tries again, and doesn't give up. But when she is with her beloved cousins, interaction comes easily; she perks up, blossoms, and it's wonderful to see her so happy, so full of playfulness.

One day, Carl, Sara, Lucas, and I go on an outing in the car. Sara is tired from all our activity and needs to nap to be able to make it through the evening. She tries to keep up with her older cousins and has so much fun that she doesn't feel it when her energy runs out. Instead, she goes into a higher gear and continues, as if she wants these days to go on forever. But she's younger and can't keep up the whole time, so the only way to get her to take a nap is to take her for a drive.

We put the kids in the back seat and drive off. We have no plan of action, just drive around a little and look at the island. Sara is screaming and angry, doesn't want to come, and doesn't want to leave her cousins. Calming words don't help, and finally she cries herself to sleep. Lucas sits quietly in the back seat. He's tired too. He sometimes plays a little with Sara and the cousins when they run around. Near the bungalow, there's a heated pool where Lucas loves to swim. The others go in too but not as much as Lucas. Jesper is afraid of the water and watches the others, while Lucas is in there constantly. Carl goes in with him and chases him around in the water, throwing him up in the air. When he lands, his head goes under, but he comes up again and wants more. His eyes are completely reddened from the chlorination, because he swims with his eyes open underwater. Now he sits in the car, exhausted and drowsy. He doesn't sleep, though. He never does during the daytime, but I see that he's resting and thinking it's nice to sit still and just relax. Sara is snoring in the back. She has big tonsils, just like Carl, and they make it difficult for her to breathe easily.

Carl and I are also quiet. It's intense, being with the kids constantly all day and, once things calm down in the car, it's nice to just sit for a while. I look out over the surrounding landscape. We're on the way up to the volcano, Teide. Its peak is 12,198 feet above sea level and is Spain's highest mountain. We can't see it yet, because it's above the clouds. We drive on roads that curve up toward the top. Initially, it's very green and we see trees and flowers along the roadside. Sometimes, a little bodega pops up alongside the road, where you can stop for a beer and food, but we drive on, afraid to awaken Sara. When I turn around and look out the back, I can see the ocean. On the horizon, I can see the neighboring island, La Gomera, but otherwise the ocean's blueness stretches forever.

We approach the clouds and soon we're in a milky fog. It doesn't take long before we're on our way out of the clouds, above them, into the blue of the sky. We're a little closer to the sun, the stars, the planets, and maybe God, if there is one. We can see the top of the volcano, which the clouds had hidden. It's a peak that rises straight up and at the top is covered in snow. The shining white snow makes a contrast with the blue sky, and I hurry to get out the camera. I roll down the window and take a few shots of the volcano and the strange natural surroundings. The closer we get, the more the landscape changes. Plant life disappears and is replaced with a barren starkness. You would think we'd landed on the moon. Lava shot out by the volcano has destroyed all living plants and transformed the surface into a stiff magma, in thousands of colors and scary forms. Loneliness dominates. The smoothness of the black asphalt road lies in stark contrast to the rugged shapes of the inaccessible environment next to it. Sometimes, by the side of the road, you can see a lonely plant struggling to survive and seeking its way through the lava to the sunlight.

Carl and I are both lost in thought, and our senses take in the strange environment outside the window.

Then I say, "Carl . . ."

"Mmmm."

"I think we should have another child."

"Strange that you should mention it. That was exactly what I was sitting and thinking," he says and looks at me with a face full of wonderment.

Sometimes, I wonder if people who live together can feel each other's thoughts without saying them, but I say, "It's probably this environment. Everything is so extreme here, life and loneliness. But, what do you think about another baby?" I ask.

Carl has always said he wanted two children. I haven't thought about it much, but he was fine with two. A boy and a girl. Perfect. However, nothing is ever perfect, and things seldom turn out the way you thought they would.

"I don't know. I haven't pictured myself as the father of three," he answers.

"No, I know."

I turn up the music on the radio and lower my voice so Lucas won't hear.

"I think it would be good to have another sibling. I'm thinking of Sara. What will happen when we die? Who will be there for Lucas? Sara will be the person who's closest to him. Can you imagine the responsibility she'll feel? Even now, when she's growing up, it would be good to have someone to share things with. You see how much fun she has with Anna and Jesper, even though they're older than she is."

"Yeah, she really is happy when she's with them. But three kids. That's a lot. It's a lot of work as it is."

"It is for a few years, then it gets easier. It's in the beginning, when the kids are small, that things are hard, but then they're more independent. It's already simpler with Sara. As soon as she's with other kids, she's gone. She keeps herself busy."

"Yes, that's true, and if it gets difficult, we could hire a nanny," says Carl.

"And think when Sara is grown up. Look at me. The people who are closest to me are my sisters, and I'll always have them. Sara will maybe never have that kind of relationship with Lucas. It would also be good for Lucas. Another person for him to love and be close to."

"Mm-hmm."

"You can see how much he likes Sara. Lucas may never get married or even have friends. But he'll always have family."

Carl is quiet for a while, then he says, "But what if we have another autistic child. The risk is greater, now that we have Lucas."

"I know. But I think we could make it work. Lucas wouldn't feel so different. They'd be able to live together when they get older. That would surely be good too."

"Autism is one thing, 'cause we know about that, but what if there's some other handicap. You're not exactly young anymore. The risk of having a child after the age of thirty-five increases dramatically."

"I know," I say, but in my mind I'm still set on having a child.

It's been a while since I began to long for another child, and the thought has slowly grown quite strong. Now it's difficult to resist those feelings. One more baby, a miracle. One more person to love. It would be wonderful. Not a day goes by without thinking of it. I'm ready, but I don't know if Carl has arrived at that point yet, and I don't want to sound adamant, afraid he'll balk. I want both of us to want this, and he should long for a child as much as I do. A baby has the right to feel welcome, wanted by both of its parents.

"I think another child would be good for our family. It would make us whole. Give us the chance to start over. Sara would love to have a sibling. Maybe not in the beginning, but later, when the baby is bigger and they can play together. And I think, for Lucas, there are only good things."

"Yes, I think you're right," says Carl.

When we return to Sweden after our vacation, we continue to talk about how we'll try to have another child. We discuss it back and forth and decide that we want to do it. It's been easy for me to conceive the previous two times, so I'm not worried about that. However, we're both afraid we'll have a handicapped child, and we'd rather not have a boy. Four out of five children with autism are boys, and that's why we would be less worried if it were a girl.

It isn't possible to predetermine a child's gender, but they say you may be able to influence sex of a child by having intercourse at the right moment in the ovulation cycle. Y-sperms swim faster and have a shorter life, while x-sperms are slower and live longer. Not entirely different from men and women in real life. This means that, if you want to have a girl, you should have sex before ovulating. By the time you ovulate, the y-sperms have died and only the x-sperms are left. I have a regular menstrual cycle, so we count the days and time our chances accordingly.

Spring comes, then summer, and each month feels like a lottery, a kind of genetic roulette that we're playing. I long for a child. I see pregnant women and newborn babies everywhere. I count the days. We plan and have "unprotected" sex at the right times, but I don't get pregnant. I've bought home pregnancy tests but never have a reason to use them, because I get my period every month. Maybe we're having sex too far ahead of my ovulation? A friend suggests buying ovulation tests at the drugstore and I try it. We keep at it and, at last, in September, my period stops. I take a test, but it shows nothing. Maybe I was too early? Too little time since fertilization? I wait a few days, take another test, and then, *then* the two lines show up on the stick and yes, I'm pregnant.

My whole body is joyous, and I'd love to tell everyone, but we take it slowly. A new tiny individual is beginning to take place in our minds, and I start to ask Sara and Lucas a little about what they would think about a sibling. Names for the child also start to pop up in my head.

In August, I started back at Talarforum again, after several years' of parental leave. People there are glad to see me, and I enjoy it, even though it probably won't be for long. I don't want to say anything yet, since the first three months are risky.

We have a friend who's a doctor. She always chooses the best health care, and she recommends that I join a specialist obstetrics clinic. I call there and ask to make an appointment, but they tell me that it's full. I tell them about our situation, that we have a special needs child and are worried about this pregnancy, and they arrange for me to come anyway. After registration, I have an ultrasound to make sure I'm pregnant. The doctor confirms that I am but wants me to come back in a week to be able to calculate the age of the fetus. A week later, I have a new ultrasound, and she doesn't think it fits with the time frame for when I believe I became pregnant. The embryo looks too small.

"Do you think I'll miscarry?" I ask.

"That could be, but maybe you just became pregnant later than you thought. We'll book a new appointment in two weeks, and we'll do a new ultrasound then," she says.

My menstrual cycle is regular, so I find it hard to accept what she says.

"Will you know then?" I ask her.

"Yes," she replies. "Enough time will have elapsed for me to see how it looks."

On the way home in the car, I call Carl, crying, and tell him I think there may be a miscarriage. We've longed and hoped so much for this child. Now there may be none.

The two weeks pass, and I return to the clinic to have a new ultrasound. I'm sitting in the waiting area in the corridor, paging through an interior decorating magazine mostly to have something to do, but my thoughts are elsewhere. I begin to prepare mentally for the worst. After a while, the doctor peeks out from her room and says, "Come in Jenny."

She's a sturdy woman, not overweight but large. She is kind and caring. I take off my clothes behind a curtain and then lie down on an examination table with my legs in the air. She does a vaginal ultrasound, because it's still early in the pregnancy. I am in a vulnerable position, but the doctor treats me with respect and kindness, and I feel comfortable with her. I can relax. I try to read her face, which is turned toward the computer screen.

"How does it look?"

"No," she says, and gives me a serious look, "it doesn't appear that it's grown as it should."

I can feel tears burning behind my eyelids.

"Are you sure?"

"Yes," she answers and turns the screen toward me, beginning to explain what she sees.

She sees an ovum sitting in the uterine wall, but it isn't fertilized. There won't be a baby this time. Even though I prepared myself for her answer, I feel sad and empty, and I ask what will happen now.

"Nature will take its course," she says. "You'll probably start bleeding heavily within a few weeks, like a period, except maybe more painful."

She prescribes some painkillers in case the pain should become too great. In a couple of weeks, it'll be autumn break and we'll go on vacation again. We're going back to the house on Tenerife, back to the place where we decided to have another child. The doctor says that we can try again when my period returns and that I shouldn't worry. Miscarriages are common, and most women have one. Many miscarriages happen so early in the pregnancy you don't even know you're pregnant. It feels really bad, like the life force has run out of me. Yet my longing for a child is still strong, and I know we'll try again. In late October, I miscarry while we are on Tenerife. Once again, life reminds us how fragile it is.

BIRTHDAY PARTY

I've been busy thinking about a new baby, and that and work have taken my focus away from Lucas and his development. At work, I've begun on a new branch of operations, arranging seminars on personal development and business with various speakers. I'm working 75 percent and taking most of the responsibility for the children, even though Carl is at home more now than before. He's still the CEO, and it demands a lot of his time. Carl thinks we should get a nanny to take the kids to daycare and pick them up, but I want to be with the kids as much as possible. Now and then, we have a babysitter come so Carl and I can do things together, like go out for dinner or to a show, or sometimes take a mini-vacation and spend the night at a hotel in the city.

At preschool this year, Lucas has a new personal paraprofessional. That's his third in a little more than a year. Toni is a sweet twenty-year-old. She has been substitute teaching at the preschool, so Lucas already knows her. We've introduced a new routine to give Lucas more time for his exercises. Every morning, Toni comes over to our place. She and Lucas start his day upstairs in our loft. They train there for more than two hours before walking over to the preschool. In this way, Lucas gets peace and quiet and can concentrate on his exercises. Toni gets coaching from the speech therapist at the autism center, and we borrow various language materials from the Lekotek for them to use. Lucas is doing much better at the preschool now. He doesn't have fits like he did before, and when I come to pick him up, he's not standing at the gate waiting for me. Most of the time, he's in the sandbox, but he's always playing alone.

The other kids who are Lucas's age have started having play dates with each other in the afternoons. Lucas has no friends; he's always with me. Each time he receives an invitation to a birthday party, I'm moved, because I know that the parents are thinking of him and want to include him, and the kids wouldn't think of it. Lucas doesn't like to go to parties, but I want him to learn to have a life like every other child, and I always accompany him to them. While the other parents go home, I stay with Lucas.

We've been invited to Will's birthday party. We walk together to his house. Before we go, I show Lucas a picture of Will and tell him that Will is having a birthday and that the gift is for him. We usually arrive last to avoid too much crowding and activity.

Lucas rings the doorbell. I take out the present from our bag and give it to Lucas so he can give it to Will. Lucas takes it and immediately starts to open it.

"No, Lucas. It's Will's birthday. Give him the present," I say.

Will opens the door.

"Happy birthday," I say, and I help Lucas to give the package.

"Thanks," says Will politely.

Lucas enters, throws off his shoes, doesn't wait to see Will open the package, and runs straight into the house toward the kitchen. I stand there on the doorstep as if on pins and needles, afraid of what Lucas might do, then I greet the parents who've come to the door. Without trying to seem unfriendly, I excuse myself as fast as I can and walk past them to follow after Lucas to see what he's up to.

He's already found the kitchen. When I come in, he's standing munching on cookies that are on a tray.

"Lucas, you have to wait until all the kids are sitting at the table! First, Will is going to open his presents, then we'll have cookies."

I brush the cookie crumbs from around his mouth, take him by the hand, and go back out into the hallway. He cries and protests. Most of the kids have run upstairs, so I take Lucas up too. All the boys are inside the kids' room, playing with toys. At first, Lucas doesn't want to go in, but I lead and pull him in with me. I try to find something that will interest him, because playing with the other kids is not an alternative. I find a green flashlight, and he's immediately glad. Flashlights are his great passion. He has a lot of them at home, in different colors and sizes and with various lamps. Unfortunately, the batteries are dead in this one, and there's more screaming. He gets angry and hits me. I hold his arms and try to calm him down.

"Come, let's look for something else. There are lots of fun things here," I say.

Lucas sees a collection of Lego airplanes high up on a shelf. He pulls out a chair and quickly climbs up to take down an airplane.

"No, Lucas, don't break it!" says Erik, Will's big brother.

"He just wants to look at it," I answer and watch over Lucas as he inspects the airplane and spins its propeller. I take down a larger plane and pretend to fly it in the air toward Lucas's plane, but Lucas is more interested in spinning the propeller on his own plane. After a while, the parents call from downstairs that it's time for snacks. All the kids run downstairs. Lucas, who's noticed all the exciting toys, now wants to stay and inspect everything in the boys' room. There's a bunk bed, and he climbs up and tries it out. I let him do it for a while, and then I say that we must go downstairs to the others.

"Come on now, Lucas. Downstairs there are cookies and juice."

"Cake?" says Lucas.

"I don't know if there is cake," I answer, because I want to prepare him in case there isn't. For Lucas, parties and cakes go together. We go down to the others, and the boys have all sat down around the table. I show Lucas where to sit. The parents ask if I'd like a cup of coffee.

"No thanks, I'm fine. I just had a cup."

I don't want to inconvenience them, besides, I don't have time to drink coffee and chat because I need to keep an eye on Lucas and help him if need be. It's important to teach him how things work at a party. He doesn't scope out the others to see how they behave, so he must be taught how to behave.

Lucas throws himself at the cookies. He pulls the Oreos apart and eats the filling. The other children are irritated, because he's just eating the tastiest part and grabbing another. I tell him that he must eat the whole cookie before he can take more, but he refuses. The parents are tolerant because they don't want any fighting, screaming, or whatever can happen when Lucas gets upset. I let him take a few more before I tell him that's enough.

"Cake," says Lucas.

Cake is one of the words he learned early. He loves marzipan cake, no others, and he only eats the marzipan. Will's mother has heard him and says, "There will be strawberries and ice cream. That's Will's favorite. He doesn't like cake very much."

Lucas doesn't seem aware of what she just said, and I hate to think how he'll react. She brings out a large bowl of strawberries and a tray of vanilla ice cream. She begins to slice pieces of ice cream and puts them on the children's plates. The bowl of strawberries is sent around the table. When she is going to put ice cream on Lucas plate, he screams, "NO!" as loudly as possible and pushes the plate away from him so that the soda bottles on the table almost fall over.

"No, it's okay," says the mother. "You don't have to eat any ice cream. Would you like strawberries?" she asks as she holds the bowl in front of Lucas.

"No!" he screams again.

Then he wants to leave the table. I try to get him to sit there a little longer, but he screams and protests and finally the mother says, "He can go upstairs and play if he wants."

I let go of him, and he is immediately on his way up. I excuse myself and follow him, since I'm afraid he'll destroy all the Lego planes that the boy has invested many hours in building.

"Wouldn't you like some coffee?" the mother asks.

"No thanks, I'm fine," I say and hurry off.

It is a difficult balance to not seem impolite, since my focus is somewhere else, on Lucas. I go upstairs. I see that Lucas is fine being alone and looking around in the boys' room, and I only stop him when I'm afraid he'll break something. After a while, the rest of the kids come upstairs. They immediately begin playing with all the presents Will has received, and the noise level rises in the room. Lucas looks around, checking things, but after a while he wants to go home.

"Home," he says.

And I have no objections. Social events in small doses are what Lucas can take and are what I feel I can cope with. We say goodbye to all the boys and go downstairs. Lucas runs and puts on his shoes and then stands, pulling at the doorknob, shouting, "Home, home." The mother hurries out into the hall from the kitchen, where she's been cleaning up.

"Are you leaving already?" she asks. "We haven't had the fish pond yet."

"That's all right," I say. "It gets a little loud for Lucas, and he's easily tired." I take him by the arm and turn him around.

"Lucas, say thank you," I tell him.

"Thank you" he says and looks at me.

"No, not to me, you need to thank Will's mom. There," I say, and point. I spin him around so he's facing the mother and I'm right behind him. "Say thank you to Will's mom."

"Thank you," says Lucas again.

"Thanks for the birthday present," she answers.

Lucas turns immediately around and begins to pull at the door again. We're ready to go out when I hear the mother call.

"Wait! You forgot your bag of candies."

"Lucas, before you go, there's some candy for you," I say, and then he stops pulling at the door. Candy is something he likes. Next time, it's my goal to stay until the fishpond, so he'll learn that activity also. Slowly, slowly, step by step, he's learning how it all works.

THE HAIRDRESSER AND
THE DENTIST

I want Lucas to handle all the situations that other kids his age manage, and I work hard with him. When he was little, I cut his hair, but now that he's bigger and is with other people daily who don't know him as well, we're careful to maintain his appearance. He already has so much to struggle with that we do everything we can to help him make a positive impression. So it's important that he's clean and tidy, has a nice haircut, and has trendy clothing.

We go to the hairdresser in our neighborhood. The first visit becomes a nightmare, even though I've found a place where he can sit on an elephant and watch a movie while he's getting his hair cut. He refuses to wear the apron and throws his head back and forth while Gun, the hairdresser, tries to work. He screams and attempts to hit her. I take turns scolding and calming him. Gun isn't particularly happy with the situation and is ready to give up. She snaps at Lucas, and, when she approaches him again, he pushes her hands away. Finally, she says she can't do any more.

"It's impossible when he won't sit still."

We pay and leave. The haircut is uneven and I have to fix it myself when we get home. In the evening, I speak to my sister-in-law on the phone and tell her about the fiasco.

"Did you go to Ulrika?" she asks.

"No, I think her name was Gun."

"Oh, but then you should try Ulrika next time. She's much better. Jesper doesn't like to have his hair cut either and runs away, but Ulrika is good. She's determined but cheerful, and she has lots of patience."

Next time, we go to Ulrika, and it makes all the difference in the world. Lucas screams and tosses his head, but she coaxes and speaks encouragingly with him, then talks about the movie, Alfie Atkins, that's showing. It's one of Lucas's favorites, and he starts to watch. For short periods, he forgets that Ulrika is cutting his hair because he's so engrossed in the movie. Then he remembers, and he starts to move his head around and grab at the scissors, but she takes it in stride and says, "Okay, let's have a short break."

She stops cutting briefly, and then she says, "It's time. Just a little on the other side. You're such a good boy. Soon you'll be finished."

She brings out the scissors and cuts a little more. I've promised Lucas that after the haircut we'll go across the street to the grocery store and buy some candy as a reward. It's important to give positive reinforcement. He says, "Candy?"

"Yes, you'll get candy after you have a haircut, but you must sit still when Ulrika cuts your hair."

Each time is a little easier, and finally the day comes when I can leave him with Ulrika and go grocery shopping across the street. When I return, Lucas asks for candy, and I reply that we buy candy on Saturdays and he accepts that answer. Ulrika smiles proudly and claims that Lucas is her best customer, sitting so still while she's working on his hair.

People treat Lucas so differently, and the way they approach him is decisive for how such an interaction will work. Knowledge creates understanding, and that improves their attitudes and the interaction.

Lucas has a dentist appointment. I tell the dentist about him, that he may not understand and may not do what she asks him to. The appointment goes rather well at first, and she gets a short look into his mouth. Then he screams some and closes it. This works for shorter and shorter intervals. To my horror, she discovers a cavity that needs filling. I ask if he can have a local anesthetic or general anesthesia, because I have difficulty believing he'll sit with his mouth open if she's going to drill into his tooth. She tells me to go to the Eastman Institute, which specializes in dentistry for children. I call, and they have time to see Lucas. They're developing a new program to treat children with autism and are happy to receive him as a patient.

Prior to the visit, I have to fill out a form containing some questions about autism in general and Lucas in particular, which I submit in time for them to read it before we come. The first visit is just for Lucas to acquaint himself with the dentist's office. The nurse helps him up into the chair and assists him in making it go up and down, lighting the bright lamp above his face, filling water in the glass, and sucking it up with the suction hose. While he's doing that, I speak with the dentist. They've designed a new routine for use when treating children with autism. I notice, though, that much of their knowledge is outdated, and I make a few suggestions for improving their routines. They wanted me to use pictograms, black and white pictures that are difficult to interpret, and to show them to Lucas before our next appointment. When I explain that we work with regular photos, they agree to my taking snapshots of them and various objects in the room with my digital camera.

Back home, I print the pictures and we talk about the visit. Yes, it's mostly me doing the talking, and Lucas points to the pictures. Before we go back next time, I bring out the photos again and we go through what he'll have to do.

Once there, he gets to sit in the chair and play again, but then the dentist interrupts and says, "Now you need to lie down for a while. Open your mouth, Lucas, so I can count your teeth. Then you may turn on the water again."

During each visit, Lucas submits to a little more of the examination. They're very methodical and take it slowly, and the dentist appointments become something Lucas looks forward to. When the time approaches for his visit to X-ray his tooth, we get to bring home the piece of plastic that holds the X-ray card, and Lucas can practice at home putting it into his mouth and biting down. The X-ray goes well, but the hole is large and the dentist feels that it's better to extract the tooth than to fill it. The tooth will fall out eventually anyway.

Our next appointment will be to extract the tooth. Lucas receives a suppository with a sedative. He lies on a cot in a separate room until the sedative begins to work, and he gets completely groggy and giggly. When we go into the dentist's examination room, I have to hold his hand to keep him from stumbling. He lies down in the chair and is too tired to run the water as usual. He opens his mouth when the dentist asks him to and receives a shot of anesthetics in his gum. It works, and the dentist can pull out his tooth without a problem. On the way home, he falls asleep in the car and I have to carry him into the house. He sleeps for many hours and wakes toward evening. When it's bedtime, he's not tired. He doesn't go to sleep until late at night, and his daily rhythm has been disturbed. It takes a few days for him to get back into the right rhythm, but it's worth it. The tooth is out.

BEHAVIORAL THERAPY— ABA AGAIN

In November, right after we return from Tenerife, there's a documentary on TV, *Cold Facts*, about autism in Sweden and Norway. It shows autistic kids who receive intensive training in Norway and are making great progress. Certain children have been completely cured and go to normal schools, without any special assistance. The program is about the same method, ABA or applied behavioral analysis, that we began training Lucas with and that I rejected and chose to drop because I was afraid we were coercing Lucas's brain. The documentary makes the claim that ABA is an evidence-based method, that it is by far the most fully researched and most generally accepted form of autism therapy, and that it has proven effective for autistic children. The Swedish health care system has until recently been denying children the opportunity to receive this therapy, unlike in Norway. Parental pressure has influenced the government, leading to the opening of twenty training spots for children in the Stockholm area. The documentary addresses the issue of equal access in the Swedish health care services, but most important for us, it demonstrates that interventions based on applied behavior analysis maximize the developmental potential of autistic children.

Carl and I watch the show, and it's difficult to deny the results.

It's been a year and a half since we broke off Lucas's training program. During that period, he has hardly made any progress in communication. Lucas will be five years old in December. Everywhere,

I've been reading that if children don't begin speaking by the time they're five, the prognosis for achieving functional verbal communication is not good, and now we are afraid that, if we go on as we have, he'll never begin to speak.

My mother-in-law, Gunilla, has also seen the program. Earlier on, she was critical of the method, but now she's been converted. She's worried, because she sees a lack of progress that she feels Lucas ought to be able to make. Soon, it will have been two years since he was diagnosed, and his speech has not developed. He uses very few words and can barely make two-word sentences. He understands quite a bit, but he can't express himself well enough to make himself understood. He works on the exercises that he's received from the speech therapist at the autism center, but we feel he needs more exercises and more intensive training in order to make progress. The speech therapist has no time to see him more often, and at the preschool his training isn't a high priority. The kids his age are developing quickly, while Lucas has come to a halt.

It's like we've been stuck in quicksand, almost sinking, while everyone is running past. The clock is ticking, and time is running away from us, like the sand in an hourglass. Soon it will be gone, that valuable time which is so important for young children with autism. The earlier they get training, the better they do as adults. We believe in Lucas, that he can learn, but he needs to be treated in the proper manner, which demands an enormous amount of effort in order to reach him and teach him. He disappears easily and loses his concentration when things get too difficult and he doesn't understand.

One week after the program on TV, Carl wakes up and can hardly get out of bed. He thinks he has a slipped disc. In the evening, instead of going out to dinner as we'd planned, we call and cancel because Carl can hardly move. He takes painkillers and lies on the couch watching TV. I don't really take him seriously, since he usually complains about the least little thing, and I think he's putting on a show. Later that evening, when the children and I have gone to bed, he's in such pain that he can't get up and come to bed. He's drenched in sweat and sits all night on the couch, sleeping fitfully. In the morning, when I wake up, I find him on the couch and help him to bed. I want to take Carl to the clinic, but he feels it's ridiculous to go in for a slipped disc, since they can't do anything about it. So, I leave him alone at home, take the kids to preschool, and go to work. Gunilla comes over to check on him and gives him food and drink, since he can barely move. She stays all day, and, while she's there, they talk a lot about the program we saw on TV and about Lucas. She thinks it would be good if we began the ABA training again.

When the kids and I arrive home, Carl's back has gotten worse. He's in such pain that he cries out when he moves, and he has a high fever.

"We've got to go in to the clinic," I say.

"No, we can't. I can't get into the car," says Carl.

"What'll we do?"

"Call Erik and ask him."

Erik is Carl's best friend. They met during military service, where both were medics. Erik is now a doctor, and we sometimes ask him for advice about the kids. He doesn't think it sounds like a slipped disc but isn't sure what else it might be and says we need to get to the hospital. Carl gives in, and I call an ambulance. The medical technicians have to carry him downstairs and drive him to the ER. Gunilla has come over and takes care of the kids, so I can take the car and follow the ambulance. At the hospital, Carl sees an experienced doctor and she understands immediately how serious it is. I sit and wait while they examine him. They run tests and then give him morphine for the pain.

Carl has a "killer bacterium," a streptococcus infection in his blood. The infection has attached to the vertebrae in his back, which is why the pain is paralyzing. His condition is life threatening and could be fatal within a few days if not treated. He's moved to the infectious diseases ward, where he receives antibiotics intravenously. He's in the hospital for a week. We talk on the phone every day. I visit him too, but the kids aren't allowed to come because of the risk of infection.

After a week, Carl is back home. He has to take penicillin for six months and will take morphine for the pain. He was close to death. We felt its icy draft and the cold chill of it. We dodged death this time, but one day our lives will end and how will it go for Lucas, who is so dependent on us? Carl and I want Lucas to be able to live an independent life long before we pass away. How else could we leave him?

The hospital stay gave us time for thought and reflection. It was an opportunity to take a break from the rush of everyday life that just whizzes by, and we talked a lot about Lucas. We both know we must do something more for him, because, the way it looks now, he's headed into his own world, which he's not able to share with anyone else. We love him and want to share our lives, our thoughts with him, just as we want to take part in his. We want to give, but also get the satisfaction of receiving.

We decide to give ABA another chance. The method is tough. It demands a lot of the child but also of the child's family and everyone around him. Will we succeed in this as a family? Last time, we had just received Lucas's diagnosis, and then I walked into a wall and into a psychosis. This will demand a special focus, an attitude in which the training permeates everything, and it demands that Lucas practice in his spare time and during all his vacations, not just at preschool but summer as well as winter, constantly.

Will we manage? I doubt that I can manage being mother and teacher both. However, my mother-in-law has an answer. She offers to work with Lucas when he's not in school. We ask her if she has really thought through her offer, and she has. Her fear is that she might put her relationship with her grandchild at risk, because there is a total and undemanding bond between them. Lucas loves her completely. However, she's prepared to risk one of the greatest sources of joy in her life, because she puts Lucas's life before her own need of satisfaction. Our gratitude is endless.

I contact the ABA consultancy firm that was in the documentary. It is a Norwegian company called TIPO, and they have recently established a branch in Sweden. I tell them that we saw the program, explain about our situation, and say that we're eager to resume Lucas's ABA therapy as soon as possible. They reply that many people have called since the TV show. The Swedish health care system has allotted only twenty spots for children with autism; they're already filled, and many children are in line. When I wonder how long it can take until we have a spot, the answer is, probably at least a year. They take our names and telephone number and put us on a list of interested families.

Wait, wait, wait—we don't have time to wait. We've already lost a year and a half; soon it will be two. Lucas will be five years old next month. Carl and I discuss the dilemma: either we wait and get free treatment for Lucas in a year through the Swedish health care system, or we pay the cost of the therapy ourselves and get going now. Counseling for one year costs more than $25,000, and that's a blow to our finances. We think that we can make the ABA work in our family, but how will the preschool react? Will they want to make the effort? The main portion of his training will be there, at least thirty hours a week. That means that the special aide must take primary responsibility for the program. Lucas will need a room of his own. The place is small, and there isn't a lot of space. They haven't been very understanding in the past. How will they be now? Can we convince the preschool to help us? Ever since our conversation with the municipal authorities, they've altered their stance and shouldered their responsibility better, but are they really prepared to work with Lucas and give him the training we think he needs? The method is contrary to the Montessori methods, and all of them are believers in the Montessori way.

If we can just get them to understand that they might change a little boy's life, we think they'd want to do their best for him. We have a meeting where we explain what we've been thinking, and, to our great joy, they do appreciate how significant the training could be for Lucas's future. They agree to accept the method and provide a room for Lucas.

I talk with TIPO again and tell them we want to go ahead with the treatment and that we'll pay for it privately. It will soon be the end of the fall semester at the preschool, and they think it would be best to start at the beginning of the next semester, in January.

SORROW

My sorrow makes itself felt repeatedly.

Before Christmas break, there is a Lucia pageant at Lucas's preschool. The children can choose whether they want to be Lucia, the queen of lights, attendants, star-boys, elves, or gingerbread men. I've shown Lucas different pictures to see if he can decide what he wants to be, but he points to them all, so I don't think he understands what I mean. I buy a red elf suit for him, making sure it's a garment he's comfortable with.

In the early morning darkness outside the preschool are rows of lit candles. The other parents are crowding into the hall to take off their coats, and the atmosphere is one of excited anticipation. We take off our coats too and continue into the classroom. There are rows of small chairs to sit on, and the air is filled with an aroma of spiced wine and gingerbread cookies. Sara is in my lap, snuggling into my arms, slightly shy around all the strangers. The lighting dims, the murmur quiets down, and soon the voices of children singing Lucia songs can be heard, then the sound of small feet on the floor. Small Lucias glide in with their crowns of candles slightly askew, followed by attendants with glitter in their hair and then star boys, with hats like giant white cones, carrying glittery stars on long sticks. Gingerbread men and elves holding lanterns bring up the rear, and, at the very end, next to Toni, walks Lucas with a flashlight in his hand. He's screaming and making noises and disturbs the others' singing, and I can see how Toni is trying to calm him. I'm sitting on pins and needles, hoping it won't get any worse.

The children form a semicircle, with all the Lucias in the middle. Lucas is on one edge, shining his flashlight. Toni sits on the floor behind him. He can't stand still. I can see how his skin is crawling, and he shoves and pushes the others next to him. Sometimes he calls out to me, and I smile at him, wave, and hold up a finger to my lips, signaling that he needs to be quiet.

The children sing many Christmas songs, and I'm struck by how good they are, how many songs they know by heart, and amid all the joy I become so sad that I can't hold back my tears. My eyes fill, and the tears find their way down my cheeks. I dry them discretely so that no one notices.

I look away, stare out the window, and see that outside it's snowing lightly. I force my thoughts onward, to banal things like what we'll have for dinner when we get home, in order to keep at bay the weeping that threatens to well up and destroy this wonderful moment, when all the parents are happy and proud of their children.

PREGNANT AGAIN

In January, Carl and I go to a conference in the Alps with our colleagues. It's the first time that we're away together without the kids. Gunilla and my mother will stay at our place for a few nights each. It feels unbelievably luxurious to travel with just Carl. To prepare the kids for our absence, I make a picture schedule of the days that we're away. I cut, paste, and put pictures in a PowerPoint program. While we're gone, the kids will sleep in our double bed, first with Gunilla and then with my mother. I make a four-day schedule. I put in a photo of our bed for each day and then a picture of the person who will be babysitting. First, there are two pictures of Gunilla, and then one of my mom. The last picture, next to our bed, is a photo of Carl and me. Each day, they can look at the schedule, and in the evening when it's time for bed they can tear off a picture to see how many nights are left until we're back.

Lucas asks about us often while we're away. Gunilla brings out the schedule, points, explains when we'll be back, and it works really well. Time is difficult to explain to children, but in this way, it becomes visually clear and they both like to look at the schedule. We call every day to say hi. We've promised to buy them presents, and Sara wants to know if we've had time to buy any yet. Lucas says a quick, "Hey!" and then turns the receiver over to Grandmother again.

We have a wonderful trip, and a few weeks later I take a pregnancy test. I'm pregnant! I don't dare hope too much, and I wait a while before visiting the prenatal clinic. We haven't told very many people yet, and I'm hiding it pretty well beneath loose clothing. This time, however, things go well. I have an ultrasound, and the baby is alive and everything looks fine. I feel a great sense of relief. Only now do I dare to enjoy the baby I'm expecting. I ask the doctor if she can tell the sex. She looks at me and says that she thinks it's a girl. I smile. In my heart, I had wished for a girl, and I know Carl had too. A little girl is kicking inside.

GETTING STARTED

In January, we begin the ABA program. Since we've done it before, we're well acquainted with the method and how the program works. Toni, Lucas's resource person, is also there and there's a lot for her to learn. It's a special method, and it's important that we note alongside the exercises how things are going for Lucas and how many attempts he needs to succeed with each part. In that way, it's easy to get an overview of what he's learning and tell when it's time to start with new exercises.

At the outset, Lucas is assessed to find the right exercises for his level. We discuss priorities and agree that the most important thing for Lucas is to work on language. Lucas has oral dyspraxia, difficulty making the various sounds, and therefore we put 90 percent of the exercises into aural and vocal training. He begins by imitating sounds and syllables in order to learn to find the right spot in his mouth when he speaks. Other children get this training effortlessly, since they naturally begin to make noises when they're a few months old. Lucas has always made very few sounds and hasn't learned any phonetics, so he sounds very fuzzy.

In the past, Toni worked with Lucas each morning in our loft, but TIPO thinks we shouldn't do this. If children are to learn their method, it's important that they be integrated into a preschool with other children. Even though much of the time will be spent on individual training, the proximity of other children is helpful. During breaks, he can run outdoors and be with other kids. Other children can also come in and be with Lucas or train with him.

Occasionally, Lucas still wakes up at 4:00 or 5:00 a.m. As soon as I hear him get up, I go fetch him and we lie down together in his bed. I lie there and hold him to keep him from running off. He screams and cries, but I want him to learn to fall asleep again. Otherwise the day ahead will be miserable. After a while, he calms down but twists and turns as he lies there singing wordless melodies. I cannot go back to sleep before he does, so on many days we're both very tired. Lucas is a morning person, so we adapt his school day accordingly. Preschool opens at 8:00 a.m., but he begins at 7:00. This suits Toni fine, since her boyfriend works as a carpenter and she has to rise early. The first hour, before the other children arrive at the preschool, Toni and Lucas train one on one, and they get a lot done.

A tiny space behind a screen becomes Lucas's very own space, where he and Toni work together. Day in and day out, they sit there and continue practicing sounds and get results. Soon, Lucas can make all the sounds, and we build on that with words and language comprehension. They also practice making facial contact. Lucas learns to say hello and meet someone's gaze when greeting or leaving them. He also learns to shake hands and wave goodbye.

One day, when we're on our usual walk home from preschool, we meet an old man who is out walking his dog. Lucas walks beside me, and Sara is in her stroller.

Sara points eagerly at the dog and says, "Look! Doggie!"

The man walks slowly, with a hunched back, and when we approach Lucas runs ahead. I see him walk up to the man, and then he stretches out his hand and says, "Hello!"

The man is a little surprised, but smiles and takes Lucas's hand in greeting.

He asks if Lucas wants to pet the dog, but Lucas doesn't dare and runs on ahead.

"Pet him, pet him," says Sara from the stroller.

When we reach the man, I ask if Sara can pet the dog.

"Sure, that's fine. He likes kids," says the man.

I lift Sara out of the stroller so she can pet the little white, curly-haired dog. He bounces around and licks her face, making her laugh.

"What a polite boy you have," says the man.

"Yes, he is," I say and smile.

Autistic children can have difficulty making generalizations from what they learn and using their knowledge in other situations, so it's very good to see Lucas approach and greet the elderly man.

Lucas works every day at school and, besides the individual program, there are goals for each part of his school day. It could be that he must sit still and listen in the group gathering, raise his hand at roll call, be able to sit at the table and eat lunch, or participate in outside activity in the afternoon. On the weekends, Gunilla comes over and works with him in the loft. He's doing well and struggles on. This time around, the ABA is going well for him and he shows no symptoms of stress, like wetting his pants.

THREE WORDS

In the spring, I find an ingenious telephone at the electronics shop, and I buy it. It's a button phone that you can program, and then you can put a picture on the button of the person the number will dial. I think it might be a good thing to have in the future when the kids are big enough and want to call by themselves. I program it with numbers for me, Carl, Grandma, Gunilla, and the cousins, then I add photos for all the people. I show Lucas and Sara how to lift the receiver and press a photo in order to call that person. They try pressing the button with my picture on it, so they hear how my cell phone rings and see me answer it and speak with them. They laugh and find it quite entertaining. We also try calling other people. The telephone is placed in the hall, and sometimes we use it together.

Before the summer arrives we have a party at work, and both Carl and I are there. Tess, a twenty-year-old woman who is a good friend of Carl's family, is babysitting. She grew up in the house next door to Carl, and he's known her since she was four years old, when she moved to Sweden from Tanzania. Tess has met our kids regularly since they were born and has lately begun babysitting for us. She's playful, and they love to be with her. She usually jokes with them, saying, "Shall we make a tiger cake?" Then she laces her dark fingers into the children's lighter ones. Initially, the kids were a little reserved when they met her, but now they don't think about it and they love her like a big sister.

At the party, I'm talking to some colleagues when my cell phone rings in my bag. I root around, find it at the bottom, and quickly pull it up to answer in time.

"Hello?"

First, I hear nothing. I put my finger in my ear and move aside to hear better.

"Hello," I repeat.

I can hear a faint voice at the other end.

"Mommy, come home!"

"Lucas, is that you?" I ask, but it's silent because he's already hung up.

It was Lucas. I recognized his voice. He's never called me before. Three words—Mommy come home. That's more words than he's ever said before. Three small words that mean he longs for me and wants me to come home, and he could say it all by himself over the phone! I immediately call the home number and Tess answers.

"Hi," I say. "I just spoke with Lucas. Did you dial the number for him?"

"No. I didn't know he called."

"Wow! Then he must've called by himself on our picture phone. Is everything fine?"

"Yes, it's fine. We're sitting upstairs watching TV. Lucas went downstairs for a while, but he's back up here again. Would you like to talk to them?"

"Yes, start with Lucas," I say. "Hey, Lucas! Did you call me?

"Hi, Mom!" he says and then I hear Tess's voice again.

"He doesn't want to say more. Here's Sara too."

"Hey, darling. Are you enjoying yourself?"

"Yes."

"What're you doing?" I ask.

"Watching TV."

"Okay. Sounds nice. I'll be home soon. Kisses and hugs."

I can hear her kiss the telephone receiver.

"Everything's fine," says Tess. "Soon we're going to bed."

"Imagine, Lucas calling by himself," I say. "That's fantastic."

"Hasn't he done it before?" Tess asks.

"No, this was the first time. Okay, I have to go now. I won't be much longer," I say and hang up. Once I've hung up, my emotions take over, and I begin to cry. I'm a few months into my pregnancy, and I'm often close to tears. I want to go home right away and see the kids. I find Carl and tell him what happened. He's just as moved as I am, and his eyes fill with tears. He understands that I want to go home and asks if I want him to come too, but I think it's better if he stays at the party. I excuse myself and say that I need to get home to the kids. I long for them, but I also want to show Lucas that what he says has consequences, that it pays to communicate.

I cry all the way home in the car, because I'm so moved that he could do something that momentous. A little voice in a telephone, yet something so big: my autistic son called all by himself and wanted me to come home. It's so wonderful to get some acknowledgment from the little person who's had such a hard time expressing himself in words.

TRAINING

It's summer vacation. Gunilla will continue to work with Lucas, so we have to plan to stay close to her. We're spending the summer out at my in-laws' vacation place in the Stockholm archipelago, the collection of islands in the Baltic Sea east of the city that's a popular vacation spot. Carl, the kids, and I all crowd into one little bedroom. In the evening, when we go to bed, we latch the door because we're afraid Lucas will wake up in the night and wander, like he does at home. It's not far to the shore, and I'm worried that he'll go down to the landing and fall in. Lucas loves water and learned to swim last summer when he was four, but I don't know how he'd react if he fell into the cold water all alone. Maybe he'd panic and not be able to get out.

Lucas and Sara usually wake up many times through the night, and it's a hassle to climb around our double bed to their bunks. I'm now in my sixth month of pregnancy. My tummy is beginning to take up more room, and I'm feeling unwieldy. Next summer, we'll have three kids, and it'll be hard to fit into our little bedroom.

Gunilla works for a few hours every day training Lucas in a boathouse down by the landing. We've moved a small table and chairs down there and made it into a classroom. We still focus mainly on sounds and words. She takes her task very seriously, and I think she feels it's a calling. She was leery of becoming a strict schoolteacher for Lucas instead of his easygoing grandmother, but it's worked out the other way. Their relationship has deepened from all the time they spend together, and Lucas loves to sit and work with her. She succeeds well in balancing demands on him and loving feedback. She spikes the training with cuddling and play, and it's wonderful to see how well it works.

Our life revolves around Lucas's training. Even though Carl and I may be doing very little of the work, it limits our life, and sometimes it feels like a yoke we must carry. We can't be spontaneous about outings and other things because we need to consider how it will affect the training program, but at the same time we know it's a small sacrifice. And actually, it's not the training that's the greatest burden; it's Lucas and his autism. Everything we do with Lucas is difficult and demands a lot of effort, and it depletes our strength, weighs on us and stifles our joy in living. It is so easy to do things with Sara, yet when we do things with Lucas we feel a certain resistance, for we know what a hassle it may become. Just thinking about it makes going out and doing things an issue.

Toward the end of the summer, when we're on the island, we find out by chance that the place next door to my in-laws is for sale. It's not on the open market, but an estate agent has been given the task of selling it to a circle of clients. Carl phones the neighbor and asks about it, and, yes, they are selling. He invites us over to have a look at the house, and we hike the short stretch over the hill that separates the two homes. The house is close, but it's still set aside. It suits us perfectly. There are three bedrooms, a kitchen, and living room. It's on a little hill with a waterfront lot.

We bid on it, but the neighbor wants to wait and see how the agent reacts, because he says he has several interested parties who want to come and look. There is a hair-raising period, when several families are bidding, but finally we're the only ones left and we close on the property. It's a fantastic place, but the location means even more to us. The proximity to Carl's parents is almost invaluable, since it makes it so much easier for Gunilla to continue working all summer with Lucas. In October, we receive access to the house.

There is a lot we'd like to do and Carl has great plans for remodeling, but the house is well maintained and functional. The first thing we do is to carry our beds over the hill from the bedroom at the in-laws' place. Then we go to IKEA and add some needed furniture. We feel extremely fortunate. Homes in the archipelago aren't for sale very often. They stay in families for generations, yet we've been lucky enough to buy the house right next to Carl's parents.

PREGNANCY

The itching begins three months before the baby's expected arrival. With Lucas, I had itching only a couple of weeks before he was born and then only on the palms of my hands and the soles of my feet. With Sara, it began a month before birth, and the itching was worse. It started with my hands and feet but spread to my whole body. The final month of my pregnancy with Sara was in the summer, and we were out at my in-laws' place. During the day, I filled buckets with ice and chilled my feet or stood and scraped them on the rough door-mat. The itching was worst at night. To stay close to the water, I slept alone in the boathouse down on the landing. Before going to bed, I would swim in the chilly water to numb my body. Then I could sleep a couple of hours before the itching woke me up again. Every other hour for the rest of the night I was forced to get up and swim in the sea to suppress the itching for a little while and be able to go back to sleep. Only the birds and I were up during the bright summer nights. Toward the end of my pregnancy, I was totally exhausted, and I begged and pleaded for the doctors to induce labor, but they wanted to wait. They wanted me to go full term. Luckily, the delivery was a week early, and once Sara was born the itching stopped.

I'd heard that itching can get progressively worse the more pregnancies you have and the older you get. That seems to be correct, because now it comes creeping in during my seventh month. It starts, as usual, with the palms of my hands and the soles of my feet, then spreads to my whole body. It's hard to find clothes that are soft and loose-fitting enough. Everything that's tight makes the itching worse. At work, it's hard to sit still, and I twist, turn, and scratch myself all over. Still, it's good to go to work because I can focus my attention on other things. Otherwise, the itching takes over and dominates completely.

Itching during pregnancy is caused by a liver malfunction, in which toxins are released under the skin. No one knows why some people get it. However, they do know that it's genetic. My mother had itching each time she was expecting, for all three of us, and I was delivered by C-section.

At the Octavia Clinic, they know about my itching, and now that it's increased, the doctor wants blood samples to test my liver. I'm surprised, since they haven't done that previously and I wonder why she wants to test this time. She says that, if the levels are high, there are medicines they can use to relieve the itching.

During this pregnancy, we're at home in Nacka and I don't have the sea nearby to cool me down. In the evenings, I take long, ice-cold showers. After drying, I douse myself in mentholated rubbing alcohol, which has a cooling effect. When I go to bed, I'm shaking from the chill, but it's better than being tortured by constant itching. Torture is exactly what it is, and doubly so. The itching itself and the lack of sleep make me want to give up.

Every week, I have a blood test to check my liver. One day, the doctor thinks it's time to try a drug, Ursofalk, that will stabilize my condition. I'm worried that the medicine may affect the baby, but the doctor says there are no proven negative side effects. On the contrary, it's good if the mother's liver function improves. When I get home, I search the Internet. My doctor is right, and I find that the medicine has shown no fetal side effects. The liver disorder during pregnancy is called ICP, intrahepatic cholestasis, and studies indicate that women in Chile and Scandinavia suffer from it most often. ICP can be intensely uncomfortable but poses no long-term risk to the mother, according to what I read.

However, the condition can be very dangerous for a developing baby, and early delivery is usually recommended. ICP may increase the risks of fetal distress, preterm birth, or stillbirth! The baby can sometimes die in the womb long before contractions start, without warning and without any known reason. I'd been told, and believed, during my previous pregnancies that the itching was only bad for me. Now I turn completely cold when I read that the baby I'm expecting might die and there's no way to prevent it from happening. I could lose my baby at any moment! I get on the phone immediately and call my doctor at the maternity center. She doesn't have time today, but I can come tomorrow.

I have to know more, and on the net I find an American site, Itchy Moms, for pregnant women with ICP. There's a lot of information, along with personal stories and a memorial page for stillborn children. The children who've died are born from the thirty-second week on until the last week of pregnancy, week 40. I'm now in my thirty-third week. I put my hand on my tummy and feel her kicking inside. As long as she's moving, I know she's alive.

I see my doctor the next day. I ask why she hasn't told me about the risks, and she says she didn't want to worry me unnecessarily. The level of bile acid in my blood isn't yet high enough to be dangerous for the baby. She wants me to take the medicine to prevent the bile acid from increasing, and to be safe I should have blood tests every other day. If the level increases, I must be prepared for induced labor, knowing that there's always a risk in beginning labor before full term, since the child isn't fully developed, especially not the lungs.

The medicine does nothing for the itching, which increases. Showers no longer do the trick at night. I fill the bathtub with cold water each evening, empty the icemaker in the kitchen, and pour all the ice into the tub. I force myself into the icy water and lie there as long as I can, until my skin goes numb. Then I sleep an hour or two until the damned itching wakes me up again and I repeat the procedure. I go to work every day, but I don't get much done.

I see the doctor the following week.

"How do you feel?" she asks.

"Well, it's still just as bad. The medicine hasn't helped at all."

"Are you getting any sleep?"

I tell her how I fill the bathtub and lie down in the ice water.

"I've received your latest test results, and your bile count has risen again. I asked the hospital, and they want you to come in."

"Will they induce labor?"

"I don't know. They want you to come in so they can examine you. There's no hurry, so you can go home and pick up some things and then you can drive over."

"Okay," I say, with my heart pounding.

"Is your husband at work?"

"Yes, he is."

"Call him and tell him to meet you at the hospital. They'll want to confer with you both."

I feel shaky. We're almost at the end, and I hope that the baby will make it, that nothing will happen. In the car on the way home I call Carl.

"Hey, it's me. I've just been to the doctor. They want me to go to the hospital."

"Oh, gee."

"I'm going home to pack some things, then I'm going straight over there."

"Are they going to induce labor now?"

"I don't know. They want to do an examination, but I'm supposed to bring my things in case I need to stay."

"Okay, I'll meet you there."

It feels good to know that the itching might end soon, but I'm worried about the delivery and the time left until the baby will be born. There's a risk that the baby will die at any time, even during the delivery. *Oh, good God, let everything go well,* I think.

At the hospital, we see a female obstetrician. She turns to me and says that they've been in frequent contact with the Octavia Clinic, and at the staff meeting this morning they decided that it's best to induce labor now, taking into consideration the effect that the liver disorder might have on the baby. It's a difficult decision, because I'm only in the thirty-fourth week and the child isn't really fully developed yet, but all the risks need to be weighed against each other.

"Will I have to have a C-section?" I ask.

"No, we want a natural birth if possible. That poses the least risk for you and your child. You'll receive something to start the contractions and soften your cervix, and that will start the delivery."

"Shall I stay here then?"

"Yep, you're in week 34, which means that the baby may be in need of intensive care when it's born. It may not, but we need to be ready, and unfortunately, the neonatal ward here is full. I've called around to see if there's room at the other hospitals in the Stockholm area, but it's the same everywhere. The closest hospital with room in neonatal is in about an hour's drive away from here, in Eskilstuna.

"That's not good," says Carl. "We have two children at home too. Do we really have to go there? How much of a hurry is there? Can't we wait a couple of hours and see if there's room anywhere in Stockholm?"

The doctor turns to me again and says, "It's impossible to say what will happen. There may be room later today or tomorrow, but it can also take many days."

I look at the doctor and ask her, "What would you do if it were your baby?"

"I would go," she answers, and that settles the matter.

We call Gunilla and tell her that we need to go to Eskilstuna. She promises to pick up the kids from preschool and take care of them until we're back. We arrive in Eskilstuna right after lunch and are received by a doctor who proudly shows us around the neonatal ward. He tells us that they have all the facilities to take care of prematurely born babies. We're admitted to the delivery ward and are sent to a German doctor. He thinks it's strange that the Stockholm hospital has sent us to them for induced labor. That's not the way they do it in Germany.

I get a room and unpack. It feels very unpleasant. After a while, a Swedish doctor comes and agrees that Söder Hospital has made a strange decision to induce labor. He takes out a textbook and reads aloud what to do in cases of itching during pregnancy. I'm close to tears when I try to explain that the latest studies say something completely different, namely that when bile acid rises to a certain level in the blood, there's a risk that the baby will die before full term. He says he's never heard of it and then leaves us. In despair, we call a neighbor who is an obstetrics specialist at Söder and tell her what's going on, that they don't want to induce labor. She says she'll call Söder Hospital and ask them to contact the doctor with whom we've just spoken and inform him of the situation. After a while, he returns and says, somewhat bitterly, that we may stay and they'll induce labor.

I receive a vagiator to get started. Soon afterwards, I begin to feel a dull pain in my stomach, which grows stronger and turns into regular pains. At regular intervals, the midwife comes in and does an ultrasound and checks whether my cervix has opened. The pains keep up all day, but in the evening, I still haven't dilated. The midwife thinks we should stop so I can sleep. I receive medicine to halt the contractions. It's frustrating, because now I want to have the baby. I don't want to wait any longer, but that's not on the table. I ask that we start again early in the morning so we won't need to go through the same thing again, and she promises that they will. When the contractions stop, the itching takes over and I can't sleep anyway. I keep getting up to shower to be able to go to sleep for a while.

In the morning, we're given breakfast, but nothing else happens. Carl goes to ask if they aren't going to start the delivery again, but the nurse he sees says the doctors are busy with several emergency cases that need their attention. The morning passes, and midday approaches. No doctors in sight. We are increasingly unhappy and have concluded that they aren't taking my childbirth seriously.

"Carl, I don't want to stay here any longer. It doesn't feel right."

"No, I know. I'll go out again and see if I can find a doctor."

After a while, he returns.

"No, there's no one out there. Not even a nurse to talk to."

I think we should collect our stuff and go back to Stockholm. Maybe there's room at another hospital by now.

I pack my things, and we walk out though the hospital to the parking lot. We don't see a single person on the way, and it feels as if we're running away. We take the car and, relieved to have left that hostile place, drive back toward Stockholm. In the car, Carl calls Söder Hospital and tells them what's happened. They're completely shocked and tell us to come right away.

During the drive, the phone rings. It's the doctor in Eskilstuna, wondering where we went. We explain that we're on the way to Söder, since they didn't have time for us. He excuses himself by saying that they had many deliveries during the night and were busy. Then he wonders if I know anyone by the name of Eva Västerman.

"Yes, that's my sister."

"She's here in Eskilstuna to visit you. I'll send your records with her, and she can give them to the people at Söder."

I call Eva. She had bought some infant clothes for preemies that she wanted to bring us, so she and her boyfriend, Finn, had come all the way to Eskilstuna.

"I thought they acted a little strange when I asked for you," she says. "They didn't want to answer whether you were here or not, and I thought that it had something to do with professional secrecy. Now I understand that they didn't know where you were!" she says and laughs.

Carl and I stop in south Stockholm to have lunch before we continue on to Söder. It feels bizarre to sit there when I know we'll soon be in the hospital again, but we feel it would be good to relax a while and eat a healthy meal before I have the baby.

This time, our reception at Söder is quite different. I start to cry when I recount what happened. They say the neonatal wards are still full everywhere in Stockholm, but now that I'm in my thirty-fifth week the risk has lessened, so we can stay and have the baby here.

I had Sara at Söder Hospital and the personnel were fantastic, so I feel relieved.

I'm admitted, get a room, and, at around four in the afternoon, the birth is induced for the second time. I'm worried that it'll be like the last time, that nothing will happen, but the doctor calms me and says that when we start the delivery here, we make sure to go through with it. There are different ways to do it. One way is to make a hole in the fetal sack, which they do after a few hours of contractions. That starts it for real. At midnight, Ida is born. I hardly get to see her before they take her away for examination and then she is put in an incubator, so they can check whether she's breathing properly. I'm taken to OR because the placenta didn't come out.

Carl comes to my room and shows me photos of Ida that he took with his camera. She is so delicate, a little chubby even though she's a little early, and she's completely pink-skinned, with a little dark blond hair. She'll stay in the incubator for the first night, but she's breathing fine by herself.

We stay at the hospital for a week until Ida gets the hang of eating. Otherwise, she's healthy. I pump milk, and every other hour I sit and try to feed her. She's tired and falls asleep. In a little medicine cup I have some breast milk that I dribble onto her lips and try to get into her a few drops at a time. Sara and Lucas come and visit. Sara has just turned four. She thinks Ida is cute and wants to hold her, kiss, and cuddle with her. Lucas isn't very interested. He approaches and gives Ida a kiss when we ask him to, but then he runs off. He thinks it's more exciting to examine all the wires and buttons in the hospital room and the breast milk pump.

At home, I continue to feed Ida with the cup for a few weeks before she can suck for herself and I can nurse her. Worries that Ida might be autistic are there from the start, and we are keenly watchful of every step she takes in her development, but soon we're reassured. Early interplay is there. When I talk to her, she looks for my gaze, and she responds to our search for contact. Since Lucas and Sara are at preschool, I have time for my baby. I was at home with Lucas too, but he was a difficult baby and we always felt so inadequate when we couldn't reach him and get a response. When Sara was born, we were in crisis, and I couldn't give her the time and attention she needed. Now, it's as if I'm experiencing a baby for the first time, and it's completely, totally wonderful. Ida and I are enjoying each other.

ACTIVITIES

Besides his training, I've enrolled Lucas in various activities in his spare time. Sometimes Sara comes along, but more often she'd rather play with a friend after school than participate in a group activity. Lucas, on the other hand, can't play with others and has no friends, and I believe it's good for him to be with other kids in a structured environment. It's a kind of training in itself.

He goes to The Little Gym, which is gymnastics for kids. It's a concept borrowed from the United States. The kids work on their motor skills, and each lesson has the same structure, which makes it easy for Lucas. They start by gathering in a circle on the thick mat in the middle of the room. They have roll call, then sing a song. Then it's warm-ups, and all the kids run around and chase each other to the tune of happy, energetic music. Then they're divided into three groups and march off to different stations where they can do somersaults, walk on horizontal bars, or do the obstacle course. After a while, they change, so everyone gets to visit all of the stations.

The parents sit outside the colorful gym and watch through the glass windows, but I'm usually inside, helping and intervening when Lucas doesn't understand or runs away from his group. I have permission to participate. Otherwise, they want the parents to wait outside. One day, a mom asks me why I'm in there, so I explain Lucas's difficulties and that he sometimes needs extra support.

"I see," she says. "I wouldn't have noticed."

I'm so used to Lucas being a spectacle, different, that it's really heartening to hear him regarded as one among others. I'd noticed her little red-haired son and wondered if he had an attention deficiency, because he was hyperactive and stood out in many ways. Maybe she was so worried about him that didn't see the other children. Parents often focus so much on what their own children are doing that they don't see the others.

Lucas is also trying out a beginners' tennis school. In a non-competitive manner, they get to learn to handle a tennis racket and hit the ball. One day, when we arrive, Lucas is in a bad mood. He screams and wants to go home. A total meltdown is imminent, and I tell him that we can buy a little candy before tennis starts. There's a cafeteria in the tennis hall. That often helps to put him in a better mood. His tantrums are difficult to foresee, and since his speech is so limited, he can't explain. His blood sugar levels have an influence on his behavior, and something sweet can get him functioning again. He refuses to eat fruit, sandwiches, and other snacks. I take him to the kiosk, and he chooses a chocolate bar. While I'm paying, I can hear a little boy behind me.

"Mommy, I want candy too!"

"No way. You know that. In our family, we only eat candy on Saturdays. No candy today."

I can hear by her tone of voice that she disapproves of my behavior. Yet it isn't possible to treat Lucas like any other child. You can't have the same rules.

After Lucas receives his chocolate bar, he calms down for a while. We hurry into the tennis hall. As a rule, we arrive just in time for our activities, since waiting for things to start is not one of Lucas's strong points. He sits in the gathering circle with the other children and suddenly starts to scream again. A tiny detail on his running shoe has attracted his attention. On the heel, there's a small loop that you can pull on when you put on your shoe, and he doesn't want it there.

"Mom, cut, Mom, cut!" he cries loudly. All the kids turn to him and some look frightened, moving away. He strikes his fists against the floor, hits me, and continues to scream. The three young instructors have gotten to know Lucas by this time and continue with the gathering, pretending that nothing is happening. I try to calm him and get him to accept the loop on his shoe, but I hear by his frustration that he won't let it go. He won't give up until it's gone. The loop is impossible to rip off, so I say to Lucas, "Stay here and I'll go get a pair of scissors."

I tell one of the instructors that I'm going to fix something on Lucas's shoe and rush off to the cafeteria with Ida on one arm, borrow a pair of scissors, and hurry back to the tennis hall. Lucas is still sitting on the floor, pulling at the little loop and screaming.

"Cut! Cut!"

The other kids have been divided into groups and have taken positions in different spots throughout the tennis hall. I put Ida down on the floor, show Lucas the scissors, and cut off both the loops on his shoes. He calms down and stops screaming, and I lead him off to a group of kids. Now I can relax for a while. I always have to be on the lookout, because I never know when something will happen and I'll have to intervene.

When the activity is over, I'm just as exhausted as Lucas is. The other parents always sit and chat in the cafeteria during the class, but I offer a hurried hello and rush off after Lucas to keep an eye on him. Ida is always with me, and, when she's tired, grumpy, and demanding attention, things become doubly difficult.

Lucas goes to swimming class too. He knows how to swim, but it's good for him to practice doing things in a group, to learn to follow instructions and take turns. I usually explain to the teachers that they need to give short, concise instructions so Lucas will understand, and it works surprisingly well. If I just give the instructors enough information, they can usually handle the situations quite well. At the swimming class, Lucas has the opportunity to shine, since he's brave and like a fish in the water. It's good for his self-esteem.

For a couple of semesters, he's also been taking private swimming lessons at the Central Pool to develop his technique. In a larger group, it's difficult for the teachers to give Lucas the time he needs to learn. At the Central Pool, they earn swimming medals each time, and Lucas had his eye on a cool shark medal that he wanted. Josefine, the swimming teacher, wasn't sure if he could earn it yet, since he'd have to swim 100 meters of both the breaststroke and backstroke, but Lucas really wanted that medal and persevered. Josefine relented and let him try. When I picked him up at the end of the lesson, he was beaming with pride and showed me his bronze shark medal. Josefine was completely ecstatic as she told me what Lucas had done. Then they continued and earned silver and gold sharks. After that, they went through all the easier medals, and Lucas filled his whole medal board on the wall at home. He wanted to earn the sea star, but that entailed swimming in the sea. I was allowed to bring one with me so Lucas could earn it in the summer at our place on the Baltic.

When summer arrives, Lucas is also enrolled in a golf class for kids. Imagine if he could learn to play golf and find it fun! That would be another thing we could do together. Golf should be an ideal sport. It's individual but still social. The swing is the same, you just change the club you use, and Lucas likes repetition. It's not an easy game, but with practice, it can work fine. Moreover, he has ball sense.

A NEW
PARAPROFESSIONAL

Lucas has adapted well to his training program and is making progress. After barely a year, we receive a spot in the program sponsored by Sweden's public health care system, which means the government will pay for Lucas's ABA. We no longer have to pay the cost ourselves. Toni is doing a fantastic job, but after a year she gets pregnant and quits. Tess, our babysitter, has been working part-time at the preschool during her studies. Now she's finished school, and we ask her if she wants to be Lucas's new aide—and she does. Tess is warm, open, and still a child at heart. She blends in well with the preschool personnel, and the kids love her. Thanks to her, Lucas takes new steps forward in his social development. Gunilla has known Tess since she was a child, and their collaboration goes well. Gunilla continues to work with Lucas on the weekends and substitutes for Tess the few times she's sick. She also works with Lucas one afternoon every week, so that Tess can have time to plan and prepare material that she needs.

When we go on vacation, Tess comes along and sometimes Gunilla does too, to work with Lucas. He's valiant and plugs on, 365 days a year.

The following summer, we have our own house. With Ida, the family now totals five. Lucas wakes up early each morning. He watches cartoons for a while, and then I make him breakfast. After breakfast, we walk the short distance over the hill to the neighboring house, where his grandmother is waiting. Sometime, if it's sunny and warm, we have a morning dip down by the landing before he starts his session.

They work each morning for four hours. Later on that summer, Lucas learns to walk over by himself. After breakfast, I kiss him goodbye, and he puts on his shoes and strolls off. I stand in the doorway of our house, with the whole sea outside, following him with my gaze. He's six years old, a little chubby and tanned, and his blond hair is scraggly after a night's sleep. He climbs carefully up the hill, disappears over the top. At a distance, I hear Grandma's voice.

"Hey, sweetheart!"

Then I know he's arrived.

When he's finished training, he wants to watch TV. It's hard to get him away from the screen in order to do other things. The rest of us are outside in the sun, swimming in the sea, going out in the boat to fish, or walking in the woods. Sara is happy catching minnows with a dip net, and Ida is always with us, but Lucas is like Ferdinand the bull under his cork oak. He prefers to stay inside and watch his movies.

Carl and I want to get him to participate more, and one day we decide that he'll no longer be allowed to watch TV during the day—only in the morning and evening, in order to try to attract him to our activities. We try it for a few days. At first, it seems to work, and he finds things to do outside. However, after a couple of days, things happen.

Suddenly, he goes into his room and I hear him crying and calling me. I run and want to go in to comfort him, but he slams the door and won't let me in. He cries, "Mom, come here!" and I return. He opens the door a crack, but then he does the same thing. He slams the door when I'm halfway in and shoves me out. We go on like that for a while, and I try to talk to him through the door, but he just cries inconsolably. Finally, I force open the door and enter. He throws himself upon me, hitting. He's six years old and large for his age, and it's hard to stop him. I want to calm and comfort him, hold him, but nothing helps and he continues hitting me as hard as he can. Then he's sad because he's hurt me. He doesn't want to and is crying again. He can't express in words what he's feeling, and the frustration is too much for him. We leave him alone for a while, and eventually he calms down. The tantrums come regularly, without any reason, and we can't foresee them.

We start to wonder if it's because we limited his freedom too much by restricting his TV time. Maybe he needs a little breathing room for himself so he can relax with something he likes to do. We let him decide for himself again, and his tantrums cease. Afterwards, we're careful to give him his own time to decide things for himself.

DARING TO BELIEVE

We've been going to the Canary Islands every year, and sometimes we go in both the autumn and the spring. The kids love it, and it's wonderfully relaxing for Carl and me. Sometimes we go with my in-laws, and Gunilla then spends four hours each day working with Lucas. Other times, Lucas's aide comes along and works with him. Lately, her friend Nina has also come, and she watches Sara and Ida while Lucas works with Tess, so Carl and I can get away and play golf.

On Tenerife, we play nine holes on the Adeje course in a beautiful spot by the ocean. Then we drive to a fishing village a little farther up the coast, where we have lunch. Boiled mussels, so fresh that they melt in our mouths, deep-fried small squid and fish. We dip the fresh-baked white bread in homemade aioli and drink ice-cold white wine. We sit right by the shore and look out over the horizon. The waves wash in over the beach, and the sound of the stones rolling around beneath the waves is a steady murmur. We sip our wine, enjoying just being there, and speak of life: how fortunate we are, after all we've been through. We're happy that we made the decision to begin with ABA again. Lucas is making progress, and we see a future for him. We have no idea how it will unfold, but right now he has a good life, he's developing—and what more can we wish for?

Tenerife has become our favorite Canary Island, because we've found a wonderful house to rent. There is lots of room and, since we always bring a large party, it suits us well. We're lucky we can afford it, but it has had its price. Carl has been constantly absent from family life. Now our business is flourishing, and we've reached the point where he's less concerned for the future and can relax, take time off. We have time together like never before.

On Tenerife, we drive to Loro Parque, a zoo on the northern side of the island. It's well kept and full of plant life. There are many animals to see, and the indoor artificial iceberg particularly fascinates the kids. It's where the penguins live. The ice mountain is built into a glass room, and snow falls from the ceiling, onto the penguins. Deep, cold water surrounds the mountain. The visitors stand on a conveyor belt that runs around the glass room. Slowly, we ride by and see the penguins standing in small groups. Sometimes they dive into the water, then swiftly glide up and swim alongside the glass wall, as if they want to greet the people on the other side.

Another favorite is the dolphin show. We arrive late, and the bleachers are already filled. Tess, the kids, and I sit down in the first row, which is reserved for handicapped people and families with baby carriages. Ida is in a carriage, so that's fine. My in-laws sit in the row behind us. Last fall, we sat in the exact same spot, and, in the middle of the show, the dolphin trainers came forward and spoke with Sara. I saw her nod and follow them off. Everything happened so fast that I hardly had a chance to react, much less understand what was happening. They lifted her down into a small yellow rowboat that lay at the side of the pool, and then dolphins pulled her out into the gigantic, blue pool. She rode around for a lap before they turned back, and a dolphin pulled her out into the middle, facing the audience. She sat there, so small and delicate, just five years old, her white-blond hair shining in the sun, and she waved to the audience with her sun-tanned arms. In the water behind her back, the other five dolphins gathered, leaped into the air, and dove, forming a dolphin arch. A buzz went through the audience, and Sara waved again, unaware of what had happened behind her. The dolphin swam back to the edge, the trainers caught the boat, and together all the dolphins swam up and lay their heads on the railing. The trainer motioned to Sara to pet and kiss them on their long noses, and she did, much to the amusement of the audience. Then the trainer with the black wetsuit lifted her out of the boat and put a yellow cap on her head, as thanks for the help. The audience applauded, and she came running to us, her face beaming with pride.

"Mommy, Mommy, did you see?"

"Yes, you were very brave, sweetheart. Wasn't it scary in the boat?"

"No, it was really fun," she said and adjusted the cap on her head. "What do the dolphins feel like?"

"They were scratchy and wet. Did you see that I kissed them?"

"Yes, I did."

So now, we're sitting here in the same spot as last time, and I wonder if they'll ask any of the kids again. During the show, I see out of the corner of my eye that the dolphin trainer is bringing out the yellow boat. Lucas has also seen it.

"Ride boat!" he says.

"Would you like to ride in the boat?" I ask.

"Yes!" he cries.

The dolphin trainer approaches. This time, he has a life jacket in his hand. Sara didn't have one last time. Maybe they've become more safety-conscious. I tell Sara that, if they ask us, this time it's Lucas's turn, since she rode last time we were here. Then I hear my in-laws behind my back.

"What if he changes his mind and makes a scene, has a meltdown?"

"Better to let Sara go."

What if he can't do it? I begin to have doubts. What if he regrets it and jumps out of the boat in the middle of the pool? What would the dolphins do then? Maybe it's dangerous. Maybe it's best to let Sara do it anyway. The dolphin trainer approaches with the floatation vest in his hand. He comes up to me and asks if any of the kids want to ride.

"Ride boat!" Lucas says again.

I hear myself say, "Sara will ride, honey."

She jumps up from her seat and puts on the vest, takes the trainer's hand, and follows him to the boat. Lucas follows them with his gaze. There is a voice in me screaming, tearing me apart. How could I do that? How could I listen to others instead of following my own conviction and believing in my son? Why should I let others' fears direct my actions toward my son? If I don't believe in him, who will . . . and how is he supposed to believe in himself?

Inwardly, I weep, promising myself to never, never let that happen again. By trying out new things and stretching his limits, he'll go further and further along and develop. I don't want the fear of failure to stand in his way. We're always coming up against obstacles and setbacks, but we deal with them, and nothing is impossible. On the contrary, Lucas and I are learning from each new situation we're confronted with.

The uncomfortable feeling of having acted unfairly gnaws at me, and I decide to set things right. We'll certainly return to Tenerife, and maybe Lucas will have the chance again. I'll do all I can to make sure he gets to ride in the little yellow boat if he wants to. Sara glides around in the water waving to the audience. I wave back and try to look happy, while I hold onto Lucas's shoulders.

He turns to me and says, "Pizza."

In his thoughts, he's already somewhere else and I hope he isn't as disappointed and sad as I am—and that he doesn't feel that we don't have faith in him.

Six months later, we are back on Tenerife. We've brought Tess again along with her friend, Nina, and we're going back to the zoo. Even if we've been there many times, it's a fun outing. Ida is bigger and thinks it's exciting to see the animals. Tess and I walk around, planning how we'll go about making sure Lucas gets a chance to ride in the dolphin boat. We don't want to say he's autistic, since they may back off, afraid of what he'll do. We agree that it's best to say that Lucas has been here many times before and never gotten to ride and that it's a dream of his.

I go to the pool alone, twenty minutes before the show starts. It's the afternoon, and this is the last show of the day, so it's our only chance. If Lucas won't be allowed to ride, I've decided that we'll just skip the show, so he won't be too disappointed. They haven't opened yet, and the entrance is blocked with a rope. I wait at the front. Slowly, a line forms behind me. After a while, a man approaches the rope and unhooks it. I'm first in and search for one of the dolphin trainers. I catch sight of a tanned man in a black wetsuit and hurry up to him. I'm glad I speak Spanish, and I tell him about my son, whose dream is to ride in the boat. He asks me how old he is and I answer.

"Where is he?" he asks.

I tell him he'll be there soon.

"How tall is he?" he asks next, and I put my hand where I think his head would be. He answers that he may be too big. He explains that it's the last show of the day, and the dolphins are tired, so it has to be a small child.

"We'll see when he gets here. Sit down over there for the time being," he says and points at a bench down by the entrance.

I call Tess and explain that it's possible Lucas won't be able to ride because he's too big. Lucas is chubby, and I'm afraid he's too heavy. Tess, Nina, and the kids arrive just before the show starts. The trainer sees them and comes over to us. I see him shaking his head before he arrives, and I understand. The dolphin trainer says that Sara can ride instead and that Lucas can come out and pet the dolphins afterwards.

I explain this to the kids, and Sara jumps up and down with joy. I peek at Lucas to see how he's reacting, but his face reveals nothing. Other kids would have been sad, but he usually accepts things if I explain the reason. I hope from the bottom of my heart that he isn't disappointed. Sara has her ride, and when she arrives back at the edge of the pool, a trainer comes to lift Lucas and put him in the boat. Lucas cries and protests because that wasn't what he wanted. Sara pets and kisses the dolphins, and the trainers ask Lucas to pet them too. Unwillingly, he stretches out a hand and pets them, and then he gives them a kiss. Both children receive yellow caps, and the trainers lift them back into their seats with us.

All I want is for Lucas to get the same opportunities as other kids. However, I don't always succeed, and sometimes I wonder if I'm not actually making things worse.

SKIS

My sister Charlotta has begun skiing with her kids. She has three children with the same age differences as ours, though hers are a year older.

Going skiing, I think. Could Lucas do that? But, of course, he could learn. It may take a little longer than for other children, but, of course, he should be able to learn. Sara is a year younger, and I don't think she would have any problems. She's athletic and has great coordination. But Lucas is clumsy and has a hard time under-standing instructions. Charlotta tells us that she uses a ski harness around her child's midriff and then she skis behind, holding onto long ropes and helping them to go slower when they ski downhill.

I love skiing. Carl and I met on a ski trip in Norway. If the kids can learn, then we'll have something we can all do together. It's easy to share with Sara, because she's so interested, but Lucas has difficulties. Most often, he doesn't want to try out new things.

I go out to buy used skis for Lucas and Sara, and I buy a couple of ski harnesses at the sporting goods store. At the time Ida is just a few months old, so she'll have to wait a few years.

At home, I show the children the skis, and they try on their boots. Sara thinks it's exciting, but Lucas refuses to put on his boots. I am unrelenting, and finally he puts them on. He cries and wants to take them off at once, but I force him to keep them on for a while and walk around in them. I've measured his foot and bought boots that are a little too large, so they won't pinch. Sara can tell me if hers are too tight or uncomfortable, but Lucas can't do that. They try the boots again the next day, and we walk out onto the flat driveway. It's a nice winter day, and the ground is covered with a thin layer of snow that squeaks under their boots when they walk around. I get the skis and help them to stamp their feet into the bindings. I take a broom, and they hold the handle while I pull them back and forth over the flat space, so they'll get used to the skis. Sara thinks it's fun, but Lucas screams the whole time and wants to go inside.

Early on a Saturday morning, Sara and I go along with Charlotta and her two oldest kids to a ski slope just outside of Stockholm. I've never been there before, and I bring only Sara the first time because I want to see how everything works before bringing Lucas. I need to be well prepared when doing things with him in order to avoid the scenes he may make otherwise.

The ski center at Flottsbro has three long slopes, and then there's a children's slope. We choose the children's slope. Phillip and Julia began skiing the previous year and can ski by themselves. Sara likes to compete and wants to keep up with Julia. I hold her by the harness, and she whizzes down the hill. Her eyes are sparkling, and her cheeks are rosy. After having exerted herself for an hour, she's exhausted, and we go to the cafeteria to have a snack.

The next day, I return to Flottsbro with Lucas. The parking lot is far from the slope, but this time I drive to the ski area and park there. We now have a handicap parking permit, which makes our life easier. If we'd been forced to park in the distant lot, I might not have been able to get Lucas to come with me to the lift area, and it's impossible to carry him with all his gear for hundreds of yards. Once we're at the slope, we still have to walk quite a distance anyway. I fetch the skis from the cargo box and unpack the car. I've brought a sled, and I load it with our boots and skis. Then I take Lucas by the hand and walk toward the lift ticket window. We buy tickets and stroll past the two longer ski lifts to the children's slope, which is farthest away. I point and show Lucas.

"See how they're skiing up there? We're going to go over to a little hill and try it."

"No, no!" Lucas cries out, but I keep a firm grip on his hand and pull him along.

The sun is shining, and I'm glad the weather's good. One less thing to create problems. At the foot of the hill, there's a large lake, and there are many people walking on the ice this fine winter's day. I see moms and dads having fun with their kids, but I'm verging on tears. Everything I do with Lucas is such a struggle, and it's an eternal balancing act to get things to work out.

On the way to the children's slope, there's a huge pile of snow and Lucas wants to stop and play in it. He climbs up and slides down. After a while, we need to get going. Slowly, we move along the foot of the hill. When we arrive at the children's slope, I remove Lucas's boots from the gear bag. I kneel down in front of him, and he leans forward toward me. I take off one of his boots and put his foot into the ski boot. He screams, protests, and flails at my back with his fists.

"Take it easy, Lucas. We're going to try skiing. It's not dangerous. We'll go together." I say, but he continues screaming and hitting me.

Now I'm hot and sweaty. I can feel the looks of others on me and understand what they're thinking. *Poor child, is she going to force him even though he doesn't want to? What an awful mother!*

I keep my head down, concentrate on the task of getting Lucas's boots on, and try to block out the rest. When I've finished, he kicks my shin with the heavy boots, and I feel like giving up, but I brace myself instead. We're going to do this, I think. I put his harness on, tie the long line around his waist, and knot it so it won't trail behind him or get stuck in the lift. I put on my own boots and help Lucas to stamp down into his bindings.

I quickly put on my own skis and stand behind Lucas with one ski on either side of his, by turns pushing him before me and stomping forward with him the rest of the way to the ski lift. It's still early so there's not much of a line.

"Now we're going to ride the lift, Lucas. We'll ride up together. I'm going with you."

"Go home, go home!" he cries and boxes me with fists balled tight.

Most of all, I want to sink down far below the earth's surface because everyone is staring, but I look only at Lucas and try not to care about anything else.

"We're going skiing now, then we'll go home. We're going to take the lift up, and when we get to the top I'll give you a piece of candy."

I've loaded my pocket with chocolate toffee, which he likes. The line moves slowly, it feels like an eternity before we get to the front. Finally, it's our turn to take the lift.

"No, no!" Lucas screams at full volume.

The lift operator, a young man around twenty, is kind and says, "It'll be fine. Just stand with your skis pointing forward."

We stand facing in the correct direction, and I have a ski between Lucas's legs so he can lean toward my leg. The children's lift is a button lift that goes slowly. The lift approaches, and the operator gives me the handle so I can put the button between my legs. The wire tightens, then it jerks tight, and we slide off. When we come up to speed, Lucas stops screaming. Suddenly, he looks quite pleased and gazes around while we glide up the hill, and I can breathe easy for a little while. We ride up to the top and get off without any problem.

"Candy," says Lucas as soon as we've gotten off, because he hasn't forgotten, so I give him a toffee.

The next step is to go downhill. I untie the lead to the harness and explain to Lucas that now we're going to ski, and I'll hold him by the rope so he doesn't go too fast. I turn him around so his skis are pointing in the right direction and then give him a little push to get him started. I follow behind, keeping a tight hold on the harness, slowing him down so he doesn't ski too fast. He has a good sense of balance, and he stands on his skis all the way down.

"Good work, Lucas! That was great! Now you've gone skiing down a real ski slope. Look," I say and point up the hill. "You've gone all the way from the top. Look, how high up! You did it! Would you like another candy?"

"Yes!" he says and receives another one. "Go home!"

"No, we're going to ski a few more times. Come now!" I say and shove him lightly toward the lift.

This time there is less protesting. When we ride the lift, Lucas laughs aloud and it's wonderful to hear. We ski down a few more times before quitting. It's best to take small steps.

During late winter weekends, the whole family goes on ski holidays to different slopes in Dalarna in central Sweden. We're staying in small red cabins, and Carl and I take turns being out on the slope with the kids. Sometimes my in-laws come along, and then Gunilla works with Lucas in the mornings, doing his ABA training. In the afternoons, she spends a while with Ida so Carl and I can be out with Sara and Lucas together. They're both learning fast, have better control, and, toward the end of the season, Sara can ski by herself down the slope. Lucas still uses a harness, but we can ski down longer hills. He loves to take the chair lift up to the top of the mountain and seems to love the speed when we ski down the hill.

The next year, we continue skiing. Lucas is improving his balance, but doesn't understand how to turn. On Easter vacation, we go to a resort in the high mountains of Sweden. Sara takes group lessons, and I book private lessons for Lucas. I explain Lucas's handicap to the instructor, that he has difficulty understanding instructions, and that the ski instructor must physically demonstrate how to do things.

In Sara's group, the instructor talks about making an ice cream cone with the skis, and I tell Lucas's instructor that it can be difficult for Lucas to understand a comparison like that, since he's concrete in his thinking. The instructor is fantastic, a young man who has a natural gift for working with children. He crouches in front of Lucas and puts his skis in the proper position to snowplow, grabs hold of the tips of Lucas's skis, and skis backward, bent over double, down the hill so Lucas can get a feel for how he needs to stand on the skis when he has to slow down. They go down the hill many times that way, and at last the instructor is able to let go and Lucas does his own snowplowing. Lucas has three lessons with the same instructor and afterwards he can snowplow by himself, control his speed, and stop when he needs to. During the final days of our vacation, we take the chair lift to the top and Lucas skis without a harness and goes down the slope all by himself. I ski next to him, ready to slow him if he loses control. I hear him laughing out loud while he's skiing downhill. He laughs so hard he's almost choking. He seems to think it's wonderful to be in control, to set his speed and swoosh down the hill. He can't turn, but he skis straight down, snowplowing to reduce his momentum. We try different ways to get him to turn, but he doesn't seem to understand what we mean. On the last day, we find a slope that's more like an access road. It's narrow, curvy, and edged with fir trees. We take Lucas there, and it becomes clear to him that he must turn when the road does, and this becomes a first step toward learning to maneuver. Lucas loves to be chased, and we figure we can teach him to turn by chasing him on the hill. When we pop up on either side of him to tag him, he automatically turns away. It's effective, and eventually he begins to do snowplow turns instead of just plowing his way straight down the slope. In his ABA training, we add words that he can use for this experience, like "go skiing," "take the lift," "chair lift," "button lift," "anchor lift," "boots," "skis," and "poles."

It takes a little longer for Lucas to learn things than for other kids, but it works. And I'm glad we're struggling onward together, because the joy of skiing offers such a feeling of freedom that it's worth all the effort in the world, and I see Lucas's enjoyment as he masters new skills.

The next Easter, we go to the mountains again, and I book private lessons for Lucas. Unfortunately, he has the misfortune of getting a different ski instructor for each lesson and doesn't learn as much as the previous year. I console myself by thinking that it's also good for Lucas to meet new people and learn to take instructions from them. At the end of the week, all the kids in the ski school have a slalom skiing contest. I sign both Sara and Lucas up. There are a hundred kids participating, and Lucas and Sara receive numbers at the back of the starting field. Tess, Lucas's aide, is along on the trip. She rides with them to the top of the children's slope, while I stand down at the finish with Ida, holding the video camera ready. It's snowing, the weather is gray, and I see them stand patiently, waiting for their turns. I wonder if Lucas will manage the course, if he'll understand which side of the ports to ski around, but I don't need to worry. When his turn comes, he skis slowly through the gates on the correct side, and when he skis over the finish line he raises his arms and cries, "I won!"

I hear the commentator through the speakers say, "And there we have Lucas at the finish, and that was the best victory dance we've seen all day. He's a real winner!"

He really is. I run out and hug him, and then we move to the side.

Sara goes right after Lucas. She comes down racer-style, so fast I don't have time to go meet her. Confused, she stands at the foot of the slope and looks for me. I hurry up to her with Ida in my arms.

"Was I good, Mom?" she says with her eyes shining.

"Yes, you were. You made it down the whole course so fast I hardly had time to record it."

"Next time I'll go just as fast. That's how you win," she explains.

Sara always wants to win, to be the best, and she wants my appreciation. I have a guilty conscience about this because I know I treat the kids differently. My expectations of Lucas are often lower than of Sara, and when Lucas succeeds at anything, he gets a lot more attention than when Sara does. Everything is so easy for her, and she has a natural aptitude for most things, which results in my demands on her being high, sometimes too high. I often give her too much responsibility, and I scold her when she doesn't do what I expect. Maybe that's why she's become so competitive—she seeks the same acknowledgment that Lucas gets when he succeeds, but to get it she has to do more.

Lucas receives a lot of my time and attention, and, now that we have Ida, there is even less time for Sara, for which she compensates by striving harder. Other times she makes a scene or gets into trouble just to get my attention. My patience doesn't always hold up, and I often get angry with her. I feel guilty for neglecting her but don't have enough strength to solve the problem.

RIDING A BIKE

Besides skiing, I want Lucas to learn to ride a bicycle. He's had a little green twelve-inch bike with training wheels that he's used on the driveway. Lucas has grown out of the bike, so he and Carl go to buy a new one. They find a silver BMX. The bar is so low that it's easy for Lucas to get on. We don't put on training wheels this time. Instead, we fasten a bar under the seat, a bike-training handle that Carl or I can hold onto so Lucas won't fall over.

I suggest that we go try out the new bike, and, as usual, I get a ringing "*No!*" from Lucas. I'll have to force him, because nothing else works. We bicycle for short stretches, just a few hundred yards to the playground on our street and back again. Lucas rides while I hold onto the bar, running behind. He starts out riding slowly and has difficulty keeping his balance, but eventually he goes faster, I can let go for short periods while he rides by himself. Toward the end of spring, with summer approaching, he rides all the way to preschool in the morning. I still have to run behind and catch the bar often because he hasn't learned to use the brakes yet. When I've dropped Lucas off, I take his bike home, get the other kids ready, and drive Sara to the same preschool. Sometimes, when Carl has to be at work early, we can't take the bike, but otherwise we try to ride the bike every day, weather permitting. Morning is the best time to get in a little bicycle practice. In the evening, Carl is often late getting home, and it's impossible to go out with Lucas when I have all three children.

There's a lot of screaming and protests, and it demands enormous effort on both our parts. Sometimes in the morning when we're getting ready to go, standing out on the driveway with Lucas screaming, refusing to get on his bike, I wonder if the neighbors won't be coming out of their houses soon to ask what's going on. I'm glad most of them drive cars, so they just drive past us quickly and don't notice how long it can take before we get going. In spite of his resistance, we plug away at it day after day, and a little at a time. Soon I can release Lucas to ride short stretches by himself. We also practice using the brakes, and, after a few weeks, he has control of his speed.

After the summer, Sara wants to learn to ride a bike too. We run along after her a few times on the street, and suddenly she's learned it. Everything is so easy for her. After summer vacation, she wants to ride with Lucas to school and we let her. When Carl leaves early for work, I put Ida in a child carrier on my back and run after Lucas, prepared to hold onto the bar while Sara rides next to us by herself. Lucas still feels unsure of himself and hasn't learned to how start going yet, so he wants me to hold the bike while he climbs on and when he gets off.

We practice one thing at a time. I try to show him how the pedals can be put in the right position at the top, so it's easy to tramp down and get some speed when starting. Slowly, slowly, in small steps, he learns the art of riding a bicycle. Lucas needs two years of practice before he's good enough to feel safe riding by himself. When he's eight years old, we take off the bar and he rides solo. I jog behind him in the morning on the way to school, and we practice what he needs to know in traffic. He must ride on the right side, stop when he comes to an intersection, and ring the bell if he wants to pass someone. When I feel that he knows all this, I try bringing my own bicycle and riding with him. The joy of riding next to each other is indescribable. It's hard to know if Lucas feels the same as I do, but when I ask if he wants to walk or ride to school, he chooses the bike.

On weekends, we often take long bike rides through the woods by a local lake, and from there to the bike path on the main road, all the way to the mall in Nacka. The carrot to get him started is that Lucas can buy a small toy or a piece of candy or something else when we arrive, and Sara can too, of course.

One Sunday afternoon, Lucas and I ride to the mall in Nacka. Every time Lucas meets a moped or a motorcycle, he slows down, stops, puts his feet down on the ground, and puts his fingers in his ears. When the sound subsides, we can continue. We ride on the sidewalk, since there is no bike path here. Lucas rides first and I follow him. A little farther on, a woman is walking on the sidewalk. She's walking in the same direction as we're riding, so she can't see us. As Lucas approaches, I hear him cry out, "Move over!"

She jumps aside, startled.

"Lucas, use your bell or say excuse me instead!" I say loud enough so the woman will hear. Lucas has begun speaking more, and it's great, but teaching him to be polite and to say things the right way isn't easy.

We continue and take the road along the lake. Past the lake the track curves into the woods and becomes gravelly, but Lucas does a good job of compensating when he skids on the downhill slopes. He's become quite sure of himself by now, but he doesn't like to ride on the uphill slopes. Instead, he gets off and walks his bike.

At the mall in Nacka, we're going to buy a Pokémon ball. He scoped it out last Saturday when we were there. Lucas likes to go around and check out the shops to look for things he wants, and the Pokémon ball was in the toy store. Most often, he wants to buy two things, but I say he has to choose one, so he chooses something and then says he wants to buy the other one next time. He likes Pokémon, Yu-Gi-Oh cards, and movies. I'm glad, because these are things that other boys his age like.

I usually give him money to pay for things himself. When Lucas has bought his Pokémon ball and put it in a bag, we continue. I want to go to H&M to see if they have some new summer clothing. I look at a few bright-colored tunics. I find a nice one and look for my size. There's a small, and I decide to buy it. I don't try it on because that would be too much for Lucas's patience. It's better to try it on at home and take it back if it doesn't fit.

I look up to find Lucas, but he's vanished. Okay, where has he gone? Probably run farther into the store to the children's section, where there's a TV. I hurry over to look for him. It's quiet in the store; there aren't many people. The children's section is empty, and I see that the TV is off. Uh oh, where is Lucas? I jog back to the entrance. I hope he hasn't left the shop!

"Lucas!" I call out. "Where are you?"

As I approach the door, I see him in the distance. He's walking up to a woman who's looking at clothes in the spot where I was before. I wonder if he thinks it's me, for we have on similar clothing, jeans and a white sweater, and we're both blond. Sometimes Lucas calls other women "Mom," and I don't know if it's because he thinks it's me. They say that autistic people have difficulty recognizing faces, even of their own families. Sometimes, when we look at photos or pictures in magazines, Lucas points to the picture and says, "Mom."

Maybe he wants to say that it's a woman, or maybe he thinks the person resembles me. I don't know for sure. Now, in the store, I see him walk up to the woman and pull her arm to get her attention. I don't call out to him but come a little closer to wait, when I hear him say, "Have you seen my mother?"

At that moment I call out to him, "Here I am, Lucas!"

The woman looks up, points to me, and says to Lucas, "There's your mother."

"Yes!" he says, smiling, skips a little, and runs over to me.

I smile at the woman and say to Lucas, "You mustn't run off like that, for then I can lose you. And you must never leave the shop yourself. You must wait for me. It was good that you asked that woman where I was. That was very well done! You can always ask someone for help. Come on, let's go pay for this."

"Go home," says Lucas.

"Yep, then we'll ride bikes home."

"*Dragon Ball Z* on Saturday," says Lucas.

Dragon Ball is a movie he wants to buy the next time we come.

"Yes, we'll buy it on Saturday, if we ride our bikes to Nacka. Otherwise, we'll buy it some other day."

He'll nag us the whole week about the movie, but that's good. Exactly like other children, Lucas nags us about things he wants. I'm happy that he asked the woman where I was. It's a huge step forward, turning to a strange person and asking for help, and he used a whole sentence and spoke clearly so she understood him.

EYEGLASSES

Sometimes Lucas does strange things and has fixed ideas that are hard to understand. Next to our double bed, we have nightstands on either side. For some reason, Lucas always wants the drawers in the nightstand to be half open. I go around shutting them, while Lucas goes and opens them and puts the nightstands at precisely the angle he wants them. I have no idea why he does that.

For a while, he would collect all the eyeglasses he could find, any. It could be his own or Sara's sunglasses, or my or Carl's prescription glasses. He would put them under a pillow in the couch, then go back and run up to the couch, jump, and came down on top of the pillow.

One evening, my mother and her husband were babysitting. I'd forgotten to warn them about Lucas's latest mischief, and Lucas got a hold of Ingvar's glasses and did the same thing with them, and had broken one of the arms. I truly didn't understand why he did it until one day when I was sitting on the couch with him, watching one of his movies. He loves animated cartoons and knows all the scenes by heart. He has many, and I'd only seen a fraction of them. The movie we're watching is about a gang of rambunctious young boys who like to play tricks on their pathetic country cousin. I watch as they take his glasses, put them under a pillow on the couch, and all sit on them to crush them. Lucas writhes with laughter when he sees the scene on the TV.

"Aha, is *that* why you put all our glasses under the pillow? Are you being just as naughty as Jerry and his friends?"

I smile secretly when I tell him, "You know, you're not supposed to do that. They can break. Sometimes they do stupid things on TV."

I go out to Carl, who's in the kitchen, which is next to the living room.

"Carl, now I know why Lucas does that thing with glasses."

I tell him where it comes from, and Carl laughs.

"Do you see how cool that is?" I say. "It's hard for autistic kids to imitate and generalize, but here Lucas has imitated something he's seen on TV all by himself. Do you realize what a giant step forward that is?"

"Yes, and it's damned funny. I think it's great he's being rowdy."

"Yeah, except it's hard to know if he understood they were ganging up on the country cousin, or whether he just thought it looked like a fun thing to do. Anyway, he imitated something, and that's fantastic!"

FOOD

When Lucas was a baby and began to taste solid food, he liked the same things as everyone else. He wouldn't eat vegetables or fruit, but he liked sausages, meatballs, pasta, rice, and potatoes. At the age of three, something happened and he became more selective about what he would eat, and his repertoire shrank dramatically. I don't know why. It was at the same time that he started preschool. Maybe the noisy lunchroom affected him, but it's more likely that his training program had something to do with it. We demanded a lot of him, and his days were filled with exercises he had to do. It's possible that his refusal to eat was a way for him to take control of a part of his life. It gave him room to breathe; he could decide the rules and only eat what he liked.

Cookies, ice cream, and candy have always found their way down his throat, but it was different with other food. For a while, he ate only pancakes, and then it was waffles. The pancakes had to be made from Bisquick, and they had to be made in a special way, thin and a little crunchy. Besides that, they had to be warm when he ate them. Since they had to be thin, it meant perpetually being at the stove to get them ready at exactly the right moment, so they were still warm when he wanted them. If they were too thick or too cold, he screamed and refused. Every morning before school I made him pancakes, and even sometimes for dinner.

At preschool, he ate a little boiled ham and chocolate breakfast flakes without milk in a bowl on the side. Sometimes he would eat a white roll, without butter or meat or cheese on it. For energy during the day, he'd have a glass of juice now and then. For a spell, he liked McDonald's hamburgers. He has always liked French fries with ketchup. Whatever isn't good for him has always seemed to work. I tried buying frozen hamburgers and cooking them at home, but he refused to eat them. I bought ground beef and made my own, and he liked those. Every week I bought a big pack of ground beef and made hamburgers, then froze them. He would eat them for lunch at preschool and sometimes at home for dinner. It was wonderful to find something that he liked and that was sort of healthy. In a kitchen supply store I found a hamburger press, and I made hamburgers on an assembly line and froze them. He also liked pizza from a particular local pizza place, but it had to be Pizza Margherita, and then, when he got it, we had to scrape off the cheese before he would eat it. For several years, his dinner consisted of hamburgers and pizza without cheese.

Lucas thinks it's fun to help cook. He likes to help by pouring cream into sauces and putting spices into different dishes. After a while, he began tasting a brown cream sauce that I often made. He thought it was good, and soon he'd traded pancakes for breakfast for sauce that he wanted to eat right out of the frying pan where I made it. With it, he would have breakfast cereal without milk in a bowl, along with orange juice to drink. He was no good at eating bread. Sometimes he would go ahead and taste a white bun or French bread. Hamburger buns would go down with the meat, but not otherwise. It also had to be a special brand of hamburger bun to be acceptable.

We always try to get him to taste different things, and one Christmas, he sampled a slice of Swedish Christmas rye bread flavored with brewer's wort. To my surprise, he really liked it. When the loaf was finished, I went shopping at another store, but it was no good. It was a different brand, so I went back to the food section in the ICA Maxi where I'd purchased the first loaf, bought several more loaves, and put them in the freezer when I got home. Finally, a bread that Lucas liked! Now his breakfast was comprised of brown sauce, cereal, a glass of orange juice, and a slice of wort-flavored rye bread—an odd combination with singular flavors that we thought were weird together, but Lucas liked it. When the Christmas season was over, ICA Maxi stopped selling Christmas rye bread. I had a talk with the store's baker and wondered if it would be possible to bake the special rye bread for my autistic son.

"Sure, we can do that," the young baker replied.

His response surprised me, because it seemed so easy. I had been prepared to argue and explain my situation, but he understood immediately. It turned out that his mother worked with autistic people.

"I'll bake twenty-five loaves and put them in our freezer, so you can come and buy as many as you need whenever you want."

It doesn't happen often, but sometimes I meet people who are wonderfully kind and understanding, and their warmth is like cotton around my heart, soft and warm. I wanted to repay his kindness, so for my part I begin telling anyone who would listen about the giant department store that could be so obliging and adapt for one small customer, our little Lucas. They baked Christmas rye bread for a year. Eventually, Lucas began to eat "regular" bread.

One Saturday morning, Lucas is sitting at the counter in the kitchen, and I'm standing at the stove making perfect pancakes for breakfast. Sara comes downstairs and sits at the kitchen counter, hair tousled, rubbing the sleep from her eyes.

"I'm hungry. I want breakfast too," she says.

"Yes, in a moment," I answer. "I'll just finish Lucas's first."

"You always make his food first! You don't love me as much as Lucas!" she says and runs into the living room.

"But darling," I call after her as I finish the batch I'm working on. Then I follow her into the living room. She's hiding behind an armchair. She sits hunched up on the floor, with her knees pulled up under her chin, arms around her legs, crying. I sit down beside her and try to give her a hug, but she pushes me away.

"Go away! Leave me alone!"

"Come on, sweetheart. Come with me and I'll make you breakfast too."

"No, go away!" she screams.

"You know I love you exactly the same as Lucas. You know that he's a little different, that he needs to work more on his Swedish and stuff and needs more help, but I love you just as much. You're my princess. Come on, and I'll make you some too."

She won't come, and after a while, I return to the kitchen. I brush Lucas's teeth and tell him to go up to the loft, where Grandma is waiting. After a while, Sara returns, droopy and flushed from crying. She sits in her chair, elbows on the counter, head hanging down between her hands. I approach her and give her a hug. I run my hand through her white-blond hair and push a stray lock behind her ear, take her face between my hands, and kiss her teary cheeks. I look into her light blue greyhound eyes.

"I love you so much. You're my Sara, my very special Sara. My sweetheart. I'm sorry that I often fix things for Lucas, but it doesn't mean that I love you less. You're fantastic, do you know that? Wonderful. I think you're such a good girl. You know how to do so many things. You're so fine, I love you so very much."

She throws her arms around my neck, and I hug her and stroke her back slowly.

"My darling."

She hugs me a little tighter. I whisper in her ear, "You're right that I always do things for Lucas first, and I'll change that in the future. He's big enough now to wait his turn."

You don't love me as much as Lucas. The words ring in my ears. Sara, young though she is, can already explain what she's feeling, and the words strike home, straight to my heart. I'm crying inside because I understand what they're based on. I don't show her how I feel often enough. I don't take time out especially for her often enough. Instead, too often things turn out wrong, and we end up in conflict, fighting. The love is within me, a natural foundation, solid and anchored within me, but she can't be sure of that. I know how I tend to hurt her, and I'm afraid it could leave lifelong scars. It might make her insecure and transform her into a person who constantly seeks acknowledgment from others, an eternal quest, when what she really needs is acknowledgment from me, her mother—so she feels loved, encouraged, and appreciated.

SCHOOL

Lucas was born in December, and, since he was late in his development, he stayed behind a year before starting school. Before we chose a school for Lucas, we went around and looked at different special schools and ones with an autism program. We saw positive programs, but also some terrible ones. One school we visited had a good reputation, but we found it to be deplorable. Without having called in advance, we were allowed to walk around freely and go into various classes. The impression we received was alarming. The doors to the different classrooms were locked, and, though an institutional feeling prevailed, it was a disorganized mess. Just before lunch break, several of the classes hadn't even gotten started with instruction. In one section, we saw a boy lying beneath a trampoline, and no one seemed to care about him. When we spoke with one of the teachers, she compared their pedagogy with training dogs.

Many of the students couldn't speak. I saw a little girl whom we'd met when Lucas got his diagnosis. She's a year younger than Lucas and hadn't developed any ability to speak. I can't help wondering if she would have been able to develop if she'd gotten the same ABA training as Lucas. We didn't expect him to begin speaking, but now he's doing it more often and life is becoming so much easier for him.

Lucas has been working with ABA for more than two years now. He's making great progress, and we want him to continue with the program as long as we see results. Disappointed by the special needs schools, we visited a regular school in our neighborhood and spoke with the principal. He was receptive to the idea of accepting Lucas and the training method we're already using with him.

Before summer vacation starts, Lucas visits his new school. To prepare him for the start of classes, I make a little book about the school. I take pictures of the building, his classroom and all the other rooms he might visit during the school day, the playground, and the teacher he'll have. I put them into PowerPoint and print a small book. We read it together during summer vacation and talk about the new things that will happen. Tess will accompany him, and that is very reassuring.

We're going to attend a parents' meeting at the beginning of the semester. Lucas's teacher wonders if I would be willing to stand up at the meeting and tell everyone about Lucas. When she asks this, the tears start to trickle. We live with Lucas's handicap and have begun to get used to it, but the sorrow over it is always there. Most of the time, we keep it at a distance, but sometimes it pops up and is impossible to fend off. She sees how sad I am and hurries to apologize for her thoughtlessness. She meant no harm, but sometimes it hurts so much to think about Lucas and all of his difficulties and shortcomings. Getting up and telling everyone about it is more that I can manage now, so I say that I'll write a letter and present Lucas that way. We believe that informing people is good, but sometimes it's just too hard.

Lucas has started school, and he's coping well with the change. He adapts quickly to a larger world. It's fantastic for us, completely awesome, that Lucas can attend a normal class. He has Tess for support, and he needs it. His intelligence profile is uneven. Academically, he's ahead of his classmates. He reads, writes, and counts, but he has great difficulty with speech, language, and social interplay. If the teacher asks him to say the alphabet, he can't answer, though he knows all the letters and sounds and can read, because he hasn't learned the term "alphabet." He's like a tourist in a foreign country, where he understands only a small part of the language.

For many years, Lucas has been very particular about what he eats and I always sent food with him to preschool. At school, they're very accommodating. The cafeteria personnel are wonderful and serve homemade hamburgers from their own recipe, and Lucas likes them. He's allowed into the kitchen while they're preparing his lunch and can help them salt and pepper it.

Eventually, he begins to try more of the dishes they offer. He tries a mouthful here and a swallow there, and now there are suddenly several things he likes. Mainly, it's the spicy meat and chicken dishes. He doesn't eat fruit or vegetables, but we get him to take vitamins and omega-3, which is an enormous step forward, since before now he has refused to swallow pills.

He has no real friends, but he likes other kids and wants to go home and visit them. He is invited to birthday parties for his classmates and his cousins. Sometimes, he visits Victor, a cool guy who's in the class ahead of him and who went to his preschool. They usually watch a movie or play video games together. Sometimes, Victor comes to our place to play. Since Lucas doesn't talk much, they seem to have little contact, but I want Victor to feel welcome and have fun here. Once, when we went to an indoor playland together, Victor mentioned that he'd like to sleep over with Lucas some time, and it's heartwarming to hear that he likes to be with Lucas and our family.

Sara has friends over often, and Lucas is sometimes included. They want him to chase them, or else they go swimming in the pool, jump on the trampoline, or have a party and dance together. When I approach them, Lucas usually says, "Go away, Mom!"

I know then that he's having fun. Every tiny moment that he's included is a source of joy to me. He has a hard time with friendship. One mother I met at a parents' educational circle told me that she'd bought a puppy for her son. Maybe Lucas can have a dog when he's older, but, for the time being, he's included in playtime sometimes and that's good enough.

Ida has had her second birthday. She's a social little person, and she likes to be with Lucas. Though she's little, she almost talks more than Lucas does. Throughout the years, Lucas has developed a love of his siblings, and he cares a lot about them. He's gentle and shows concern when, for example, they fall and hurt themselves. Like all children, they quarrel and fight sometimes, but he shows great regret when he's done something thoughtless and can begin to cry if he's hurt one of them. Lucas is a kindhearted person who cares about others. If one of us is away, he wants to know where they are and when he or she will be back home again. He wants the family to be together. He's like a shepherd who wants to keep the flock, us, together. Sometimes, he makes small drawings with stick figures of the members of our family, prints our names beneath each figure, and puts it up on the wall.

I'm glad we have a big family—that we decided to have another child. Lucas and Sara love Ida. All three are so different, but they like each other anyway.

They all sleep in the same room. We've put two twin beds together to make a double bed, and they all sleep there together. They sleep better that way. If they wake up at night, they feel safety in the closeness, and then they drop back to sleep.

One evening, I'm reading a story to the children. Ida and Sara fall asleep before it's over, but Lucas is still awake. I finish reading, kiss him good night, and get up to go.

Then Lucas says, "Mommy, stay here."

"Do you want me to lie next to you?"

"Yes!" he says eagerly, with a voice full of joy.

My heart melts, and I lie down next to him again. When he was younger, he didn't like to be close, but now he thinks it's cozy. We spoon, and his soft body is completely relaxed.

It's late, and it's gotten dark out. Thunderstorms have been in the air all evening, and suddenly a bolt of lightning pierces the window and the curtain, lighting up the room. Then we hear the rumble.

"Mommy, monster out there," he says. "Hide under blanket!"

He disappears beneath the covers.

"Come on, Mommy!" I hear him whisper.

I crawl in after him and pull the blanket over our heads.

"It's just the thunder, dear. There are no monsters or ghōsts. They're only in movies and books. Just pretend. What does Alfie Atkins usually say to them?" I ask him.

"Be gone, you nasty ghost, 'cause you're not real."

"Yes, that's right. They're not real."

We lie there, holding each other in the warmth of the blanket. The rains taps on the windowpane, and the wind wails in the treetops. After a while, we emerge and lie properly. I have my arm around his waist and am cuddling up to his neck. Then I hear how his breathing slows, and he falls asleep. I must have dozed off, because, in the middle of the night, Lucas awakens me.

"Mommy?" he calls anxiously.

I search for him, stretch out my hand, and hold him.

"I'm here, dear. Go back to sleep now," I say, groggy.

He moves close to me, and I can feel him grab a lock of my hair and begin to twist it around his finger. I stop him and take his hand away, so my hair won't get snarled and full of small knots. He twists and turns on the bed for a while before he calms down. We lie still next to each other in the dark, but I can hear that he's awake. He lies quietly for a long while. Then he says, clearly and concisely, "Mommy, it's stopped raining now."

Yes, my darling, I think. *You're right. Now it's stopped raining.*

AFTERWORD

Today Lucas is sixteen years old. He went to a regular school up until sixth grade. After that he started in a school for children with special needs.

Like many parents of children with autism, we had dreamed that our son would overcome his diagnosis. Lucas still has autism, but despite this, he has matured and developed amazingly, and we're so proud of him. He is such a loving, kind, and generous individual, and if everyone were like him, the world would be a more peaceful place.

We have continued training with ABA, which laid the groundwork for his language and other skills. We have always included him in our life just as much as his siblings, and because of that he's used to many situations and has also developed independence. He rides his bike or takes the commuter train to school. He goes swimming, shopping, dines, and goes to the movies with friends.

In 2013 we moved to the United States. The transition has gone well, and Lucas is now attending school here and learning English. He has downloaded the Google Translate app on his iPhone and uses it frequently. His vocabulary is expanding, and it's incredible to see how he's able to cope in this new environment. He loves playing video games and watching movies, often in English but also in Spanish! And then his iPhone app really comes in handy.

Recently, we got a Lab puppy named Titus, and the bond developing between them is wonderful to watch. Titus completely admires Lucas. It's adorable to see how happy he is when Lucas is around, and for his part, Lucas is learning a lot from the puppy, watching and interpreting his body language and connecting with him. Lucas's communication skills have improved even more, and it's so sweet seeing a deep relationship forming between them. I think Lucas will have a very loyal and loving companion for many years to come.

ACKNOWLEDGMENTS

I dedicate this book to my mother-in-law. She is the one who has taken the most responsibility for our son's training. In doing so, she placed the unconditional love of her grandchild at risk, but she put his development before all else. Much to our joy, their relationship has deepened from all the time they've spent together. My mother-in-law is an outstanding person, and we're lucky to have her in our lives.

Thanks also to all the other people—therapists, teachers, doctors, relatives, and friends—who meet our son with an open mind, who encounter him with love, warmth, and respect. You must know that you're important. You're making a huge difference in his life.